Understanding and Supporting Professional Carers

Janet Thomas

Independent counsellor for work-related stress, health concerns and relationships

Foreword by
Michael Carroll

Radcliffe Publishing
Oxford • Seattle

Radcliffe Publishing Ltd
18 Marcham Road
Abingdon
Oxon OX14 1AA
United Kingdom

www.radcliffe-oxford.com
Electronic catalogue and worldwide online ordering facility.

British Library Cataloguing in Publication Data

A catalogue record for this book is available from the British Library.

ISBN-10 1 85775 798 X
ISBN-13 978 1 85775 798 9

Typeset by Anne Joshua & Associates, Oxford
Printed and bound by TJ International Ltd, Padstow, Cornwall

Contents

Foreword

In a number of professions the instrument that gets the work done is the person him or herself. Practice is more than simply the application of knowledge or skills. Emerson put it well when he wrote, 'What you *ARE* shouts so loudly in my ears I cannot hear what you say' and Stephen Covey makes a similar point, 'You *ARE* the message'.[1] Parents are more than people who pass on information and competencies to their children. Who they are, what values they hold and how they relate to their offspring are more important than anything they say or the knowledge they have. They themselves are the tools of their trade.

Stephen Covey called this 'sharpening the saw'. If the saw earns you your livelihood then make sure it is sharp. If you are the medium of your helping then ensure you are in peak condition. Look after yourself. As a wise Maori shared with me last year, 'When I am well, my clients are well'. Earlier Carl Rogers had summarised the same sentiments when he indicated that changes in him brought about amazing changes in others.

Sports psychology and sports studies have also been instrumental in helping us understand that behind performance is energy: physical energy, emotional energy, mental energy and spiritual energy. These four types of energy become crucial to athletes remaining in excellent condition. All four are needed, not just one on its own. Physical energy is the amount of our energy; emotional energy is the quality of our energy; mental energy is the focus of our energy and spiritual energy is the source of our energy. If all four types of energy are necessary to keep sports men and women at their best, then, even more so, they are needed for employees who engage in demanding jobs. *The Corporate Athlete*[2] is the title of a book translating this knowledge from sports studies into the corporate world. It asks: 'How does the corporate athlete stay energised, focused, motivated and giving excellent service?' A similar question is the essence of *Understanding and Supporting Professional Carers*: how can professional carers stay psychologically and emotionally healthy while engaged in demanding jobs?

All this leads to a simple truism – if you do not look after yourself then your work will suffer. It also connects to organisations and institutions – if you do not look after your employees, their work will suffer.

A healthy workforce in the helping professions is the subject of this book by Janet Thomas. Her focus is the one above – how can we understand and support professional carers? This is not a new subject and the stresses of professionals in the helping professions are well documented. However, what Janet does well is gather a lot of material together in one place and weave it into a valuable summary of how to understand and support professional carers. There are up-to-date statistics, there are pertinent and widespread examples, there is a comprehensive list of strategies for supporting professional carers and there is a systemic understanding of the roots of stress for practitioners in the helping professions.

Janet is keen to support a systemic view in making sense of and providing support for carers. It is too easy to blame, to find a single cause, to be simplistic about solutions. Blame the organisation; make the individual responsible for himself/herself. Janet does not do that. She looks inside the professional to articulate how personality, motivation and rationales for choosing their vocations can impact on stress: she looks outside to see how organisational culture and organisational strategies can influence the mental well being of employees. It is neither one nor the other, both need to be kept in mind: there is 'compulsive caring' and there are organisational structures that stress.

Reading this book reminded me of putting together a jigsaw. Janet's book patiently takes the pieces and, in a slightly hidden way, begins to fit them together: suddenly, the big picture emerges. The final message is not hard to understand: 'Ultimately, understanding and looking after the welfare of the workforce lead to a happier, healthier and more effective service' (*see* Introduction). Excuse the mixed metaphors but that's both the big picture and the book in a nutshell.

Michael Carroll
Visiting Industrial Professor
University of Bristol
August 2006

References

1 Covey S (1989) *The Seven Habits of Highly Effective People*. Simon and Schuster, London.
2 Groppel J (2000) *The Corporate Athlete: how to achieve maximal performance in business and life*. Wiley, New York.

Preface

This book was born out of the ongoing and probably inevitable struggle to reconcile the caring aspects of health and social care with the need for control of economic and emotional resources. It reflects a journey I have made in my own career. I was a doctor, a professional carer, and I quickly discovered that my professional colleagues often had ongoing emotional difficulties. Many became disgruntled or even disillusioned when they found that their work did not result in the expected job satisfaction. Others were unhappy for less obvious reasons, perhaps to do with unconscious personal conflicts. Some found that their commitment to their work had a detrimental effect on their marital and family relationships. Most had never considered the organisational restrictions of a career as a professional carer.

In the light of my experience as an informal counsellor and later a Relate counsellor, I eventually decided to train as a professional counsellor. Working as a counsellor for hospital and local government staff has given me further insight into the organisational and administrative aspects of health and social care. I offer these insights to those who work in health and social services, especially those who care about the well-being and performance of employees. Managers at all levels of the hierarchy, human resource officers, workplace counsellors and supervisors will all find useful information in this book. Professional carers who want to understand themselves better and gain more satisfaction from their work will also find it illuminating.

In order to be able to help staff effectively, it is necessary to be able to see the problems from both sides of the fence. It is pointless to focus only on the personal aspects of a problem. Although the organisation is not present in the counselling room, it is metaphorically present, like the proverbial elephant in the corner. Managers and counsellors must consider the whole system when unravelling staff problems, otherwise it is impossible to develop lasting and effective interventions.

All those who work in the caring professions try to meet the needs of their patients and clients in a sensitive way, within the limitations of their own emotional stamina and the practical and financial constraints of the employing organisation. They often struggle in private with these conflicting values because they seem to have nowhere to explore their feelings. They may perceive that no one will understand them, or that they are peculiar in some way. The value of providing a staff support service is that this gives people permission to ask for help, and it provides a safe place in which to explore and resolve stress. More and more health and social care professionals are starting to use support services, and as a result of their positive experience of staff support, are recommending such services to others.

Patients and clients are often vulnerable because of ill health or social deprivation, and may sometimes seem to make unreasonable demands on professional carers. This puts an additional strain on the professionals who are helping them. If the professionals are also vulnerable, the task may become unmanageable. In the first chapter of the book I explore some of the psychological reasons for emotional vulnerability in health and social care professionals. Often these are connected to the original underlying motivation for their choice of career.

It is equally important to understand the organisational and managerial aspects of health and social care, because these contribute to the tension between overwhelming demand and economic restraint. Many managers and politicians have tried to solve these problems. If it were easy, we would have a solution by now. Frequent political initiatives and organisational changes are evidence that there is no easy answer. Every twist and turn causes further harassment for managers, professionals and service users.

I do not have the solution either, but I believe that an understanding of the psychological and organisational processes can result in more effective staff support, greater satisfaction for professionals and thus a better service for the public. The chapter on the effects of stress on staff indicates that these are not trivial problems. The damage to individuals' emotional health and the resulting poor performance and sickness absence have a major impact on service delivery. The examples that I give show that there are many interventions which can make a difference. The range of staff support available indicates that help can be tailored to the needs of different organisations and a variety of situations.

In the end, the book is about optimism. Understanding and accepting reality frees us to work with the problems rather than having to fight the inevitable.

All through the book I give examples based on my own experience, including details of the interventions that made a difference. Clients have given express permission for me to use this information. However, I have protected client confidentiality by changing many details. Readers will notice that I have used the female gender throughout the book, except in some of the case examples. Many carers, managers and counsellors are female, but of course men do these jobs as well. I have merely tried to avoid confusion by choosing one form of pronoun. The casework examples confirm that men and women are equally likely to be affected by the stresses described.

Janet Thomas
August 2006

About the author

Janet Thomas started her professional life as a doctor, training at the Royal Free Hospital School of Medicine in London. At that time, 'The Free' was unique in promoting women in medicine, and was a long way ahead of the field in fighting for sexual and racial equality.

After completing her basic training, Janet chose to specialise in haematology. This entailed several years of postgraduate training to gain membership of the Royal College of Pathologists and the British Society for Haematology. As she developed professionally, the specialty was also undergoing a process of dramatic change, as a result of the rapid advancement of knowledge about leukaemia and other blood diseases. This was her first taste of the ongoing process of change within the NHS. She realised that change was inevitable and that it was important to work with it rather than try to fight it. Embracing change has enabled her to progress in her career and grasp new opportunities.

The opportunity to train as a counsellor emerged from her realisation that many of her haematology patients wanted to talk about their illness and understand the choices available to them. She also found that her colleagues wanted to talk about their problems and would seek out a quiet time to bend her ear. She decided to train as a Relate counsellor. At the time she could not manage a diploma course, due to family and work commitments, so the Relate system of weekend school suited her. She worked as a voluntary counsellor for Relate for many years, and she also ran a vocational counselling scheme for junior doctors in the hospital where she worked.

Eventually Janet decided that she was more of a counsellor than a doctor, so she retired from haematology and started a private practice in counselling. She gained accreditation from the British Association for Counselling and Psychotherapy. Although she continues to work with couples, her work now includes the problems of the relationship between workers and their work, especially in the field of health and social care. Her special interest is informed by the fact that she has been on both sides of the fence – she was a healthcare professional, and now she is a healthcare counsellor.

Family life has always been important to her. The values she absorbed in childhood were about the importance of family support, good health and education, and all of these continue to matter to her. Education was the key to advancement, and Janet's parents made sure that she had the chance to benefit from this. She has done the same for her children. Now she has knowledge and experience that she can share for the benefit of her fellow professionals. She knows from personal experience the value of a supportive family, understanding colleagues and the availability of another layer of professional help.

Acknowledgements

The inspiration for this book comes from my own experience of working in a hospital staff counselling service. During the process of counselling, my clients have trusted me with their experience and given written permission for me to use this information without identifying individuals. I am deeply indebted to all my clients. Each of them has added to my knowledge, and I have used this knowledge to help others and to write this book.

My husband, David, has helped me to develop my ideas, and he has been constantly and patiently available as my technical expert. I am grateful to all my colleagues, who have shared their ideas, supported my counselling and loaned books to help my research. In particular, Jan Clarke, Caroline Pullen, Rosie Spurr and Christine White have always been encouraging and willing to give critical feedback. Rita Lees, Carolyn Lewis, Elspeth Schwenk and Geraldine Taylor encouraged me to believe in the possibility of writing a book, and have been generous with their support. Margaret Pettifer has been inspirational and generous with her time, and tolerant of my inexperience as a writer.

Thank you to everyone for making it possible for me to write this book.

Introduction

Health and social care affect the life of everyone. The focus for professional caring is its effect on those who are the recipients of care, but we must also pay attention to the personnel who provide that care. Increasing our understanding of why people choose to work in the caring professions, and of the culture of these organisations, enables us to address some of the stress and unhappiness that lead to illness, disillusionment and discontent among professional carers.

This book is for those who work in the health service, social work, the professions allied to medicine and the voluntary sector, including their managers, personnel officers and counsellors. Ultimately, understanding and looking after the welfare of the workforce lead to a happier, healthier and more effective service.

I have drawn extensively on my many years' experience both as an employee and as a counsellor for the National Health Service (NHS). My personal journey to becoming a professional carer started with gradual conditioning throughout my childhood. My mother was the family carer, and she was always ready to offer help and support to friends and neighbours who had problems. As quite a small child I recall a sense of her pity for people who were ill. Diseases such as polio and scarlet fever occurred among my friends, and we were thankful to be spared these. The subliminal message was 'Our family is strong and healthy.' My older sister became a nurse. We were proud of her achievement of a professional career in caring that also brought opportunities to travel and work abroad.

My school assumed that I would follow family tradition and train to be a nurse, but I had higher ambitions to study medicine at university. Perhaps I was spurred on by a rebellious streak or competition with my peers. Medical training was very arduous for me, and I found caring for patients very stressful. To my surprise the staff seemed to have at least as many problems as the patients.

As my career developed I found that colleagues had a habit of seeking my support in times of stress. I also gained a reputation for being sympathetic and approachable in my clinical work. Patients have subtle ways of getting what they want from the NHS. Outpatient clinics may often seem to be badly organised, but the disorganisation allows patients to manipulate the system so that they are often able to see the doctor who best suits them. In my experience the patients who wanted time to talk over their fears and explore their treatment options would ask to see me, whereas the patients who wanted a detailed exposition of the latest research chose another colleague.

Eventually I came to the conclusion that I should undertake counselling training. I had become a counsellor by stealth and now needed to learn how to do it properly. The boundaries between sympathetic advice and counselling were blurred and had to be re-established in a more professional way. I was able to set up a formal vocational counselling service for junior doctors, and I later joined the hospital staff counselling service as an associate counsellor. Instead of being a doctor, I am now a counsellor. My understanding of the problems encountered by professional carers is underpinned by my own learning and experience.

The format of this book follows a similar pattern. I explore the conscious and unconscious reasons why people choose health and social care as an occupation. The chapters on organisational culture look at hierarchy, systems, organisational change and professional standards. These all have an impact on individual workers. The mismatch between the aspirations of the carers and the requirements of the organisation, patients and clients sets the scene for work-related stress.

The symptoms and signs of stress are explained in the context of professional caring. I use case studies to illustrate the ways in which distressed workers may present themselves for help. Clients have given permission for me to do this, but the details have been changed to ensure anonymity. If any of the stories seem familiar to you, it is because they are all frequent scenarios that represent recurring problems in health and social care. Helpful and sometimes unhelpful interventions described in the case reports will help practitioners and managers to improve their own performance.

Recognition of stress in the workplace is now embedded in employment practice, and legal precedents have been set for the provision of support for employees who are experiencing work-related stress. This provision can be made in various ways. The final chapter explores the range of staff support services available. In addition to employee counselling programmes, most professional carers will have a number of opportunities to obtain help – from personal insight, peer and managerial support, their union or professional body and services available to the general public through health and voluntary providers.

Managers and human resource officers will find it helpful to understand how overt and subconscious impulses specific to health and social care may affect employees' motivation and effectiveness. Perhaps you are a counsellor working for staff support services in health and social care settings. You will already be facing the issues I describe and will gain new insight. Counsellors in private practice often have clients who work in health and social care, and will be able to learn more about the impact that the client's occupation has on her emotional life. You may be an emotionally aware person working in this type of job and keen to learn more about yourself. This book will help you to gain insight into your own motivation and stress reactions.

My aim is to normalise the professional carer's need for self-monitoring, personal growth and appropriate support. Caring is rewarding, stressful and important work. We should value what we do, and allow ourselves to recognise that from time to time the emotional scales need to be rebalanced. Professional carers, managers, human resource personnel and counsellors will all find useful information in this book that will enable them to be happier and more successful in their work and personal life. I hope that by sharing my experience I can help, inspire and inform others to continue the work of caring.

I have used the female gender in the text, except for case histories of male workers. This is for simplicity, but I recognise that many doctors, nurses, social workers, managers and counsellors are men, and your work is valued every bit as much as that of women.

Chapter 1

The relationship between personality and career choice

Introduction

The provision of staff support and counselling services for those who work in health and social care has evolved from recognition that these are stressful jobs. The personal factors in work-related stress in health and social care will be explored in this chapter, while Chapters 2 and 3 explore the contribution of organisational issues to the stress equation.

Many people have a vocation to do this challenging work. Often they know why they have made their choice, but sometimes there are hidden incentives. This chapter examines some of the possible conscious and unconscious reasons why doctors, nurses, social workers, counsellors and allied professionals join the caring professions.

The conscious reasons include practical considerations such as training, income and widespread availability of work. Family tradition has a strong influence on career choice, but not only in the caring professions. Some see caring as a worthwhile and satisfying job that helps to make a difference to people's lives. Others gain a sense of belonging or importance from being part of a respected profession with a strong, sometimes uniformed, identity. Social workers may have a conscious desire to rectify unfairness and deprivation.

When asked why they have entered the medical profession, many nurses and doctors answer 'I want to make people better.' Sometimes they do not know the answer to this question and may say, for example, 'I have always wanted to be a nurse.' Allen[1] found that many doctors had never seriously considered any other career. These answers indicate that career decisions were made very early on, and that subconscious factors from early childhood probably influenced their choice. Childhood events sometimes remain unresolved until adult life, when life choices might be aimed at reparation or resolution. Choosing to pursue a career in health or social care is one way to achieve this self-satisfaction.

Because of the subconscious element in career choice, it may not be obvious why people sometimes become disillusioned with their work. When workers are unhappy, stressed or unsuccessful in their job, managers and counsellors are more likely to be able to help them if they understand the underlying issues. I hope that these ideas will also be enlightening for carers who want to know themselves better and become more effective in their work.

Conscious choice

Health and social care is a very large employment sector that offers opportunities to workers at all levels, including highly skilled professionals, technicians, administrators, and care workers who need few qualifications. It is likely that many will choose to work in these settings for purely practical reasons. Secure employment in a convenient location may be sufficient to fulfil their needs.

If a person discovers that she has a natural aptitude for looking after people, she may consciously seek to work in a caring capacity in order to make use of her ability. People with a variety of skills may feel that they want to use those skills in a way that helps others. 'I want to work with people' is a frequently quoted reason, implying that many people enjoy human contact. For instance, a physicist may get more immediate satisfaction from working in a hospital radiotherapy department, where she can see patients directly benefit from her expertise, than if she worked in an academic research institute where the value of the work is less visible.

Medicine is one of the careers that require an understanding of science. Allen[1] found that, among the young doctors she interviewed in 1986, nearly a quarter of the men and over one-fifth of the women had decided to study medicine because they were good at science subjects at school. Other reasons given in this survey included a perception that medicine is a good and worthwhile career, or to fulfil the aims and aspirations of others.

Careers advice

Justin, a talented boy, was exploring his career options before entering the sixth form at his school. He was particularly bright at chemistry, and decided that he would like to pursue a career in biochemistry. The careers master encouraged him to look at medical biochemistry, and told him that if he chose this career his prospects would be far better if he trained as a doctor and later specialised in biochemistry.

This advice worked out well for Justin, as he became a successful hospital biochemist. He also enjoyed higher status and greater earning potential in the medical profession than he might have had as a non-medical scientist.

Altruism

Unselfish concern for the welfare of others underpins care work and is an important factor for many voluntary workers. However, altruism may not be all that it seems. The rewards may include a salary, public approval and the satisfaction of meeting others' needs. The invisible reward is the meeting of the worker's psychological needs. In this sense it is closely linked to compulsive caring, which is explored later in this chapter. Compulsive carers care for others in order to satisfy their own psychological inadequacy. An altruist is able to tolerate the emotional imbalance of a caring role so long as she has other sources of ego satisfaction to compensate. The emotional energy expended on looking after others may be restored by praise from colleagues, friends and family, or by other recreational activities. In other words, altruists keep a balance in their life by developing ways of looking after themselves emotionally.

Financial rewards do not always reflect the importance of work in health and social care, and there may be an assumption that the feeling of doing a worthwhile job will compensate for this. Employers sometimes consciously or unconsciously exploit altruistic workers' goodwill. In the helping professions there is sometimes a sense of moral obligation to do more than the minimum laid down in the job description. Nurses working on understaffed wards find it hard to leave patients untended if their shift finishes and there is no one to take over their unfinished tasks. They may skip meal breaks because they don't have time to stop what they are doing.

Recognition that workers are being exploited in this way is slowly gaining ground, but working to rule or campaigning for fairer conditions gives a bad impression. A nurse may feel that she would lose public respect if she held out for better pay and conditions, whereas such behaviour is held to be acceptable for other occupations. It is common for care workers to absorb overload and keep on coping until they are unable to do so any longer. When stress or illness overtakes them they are forced to stop, and they may be unable to return to work for weeks or months, or sometimes not at all.

A bad back

Carol described an insidious build-up of work to meet ever-increasing targets until she eventually went off sick with backache. She was not the only person on the ward to feel the strain – others had also had periods of sick leave. When colleagues were off sick, the workload continued and the rest of the team was expected to take up the work, thus becoming progressively more overloaded and vulnerable to illness.

Carol's recovery programme included exercises for her back pain. She also decided to work on an assertiveness course that involved learning to say 'no' to unreasonable requests. She admired the way some of her colleagues were able to do this, and proceeded to learn how to do so herself. In this way she was able to protect herself from relapse of her pain. She learned that altruism does not include having to say 'yes' to all demands. When she became more assertive, she was able to conserve her emotional and physical strength, and she became more effective in her work.

Doctors also sometimes have difficulty saying 'no' to overwork. Until recently many hospital doctors had a 'whole-time' contract with no specified hours of work. In 1995 it was agreed that junior doctors should not work more than an average of 56 hours per week (or 72 hours in less pressurised jobs), but many doctors still work more than the agreed limit.

In reality the work is never done. There is no point at which the medical in-tray is empty, so each doctor must learn to set their own boundaries. When I worked as a vocational counsellor for junior doctors, I would see a succession of newly qualified doctors every six months to explore their career concerns. With each six-month block the nature of the job would remain the same, but I was struck by how differently the individuals perceived the job. One doctor would say 'I'm really loving it, it's busy but I can cope with that', while another would say 'I'm totally overloaded, I don't know how I'm going to get through this.' Some managed to finish work at a reasonable time, but others regularly stayed on the wards late into the evening.

At this stage in their careers many had yet to learn how to manage their time. The highly conscientious and the perfectionists sometimes set themselves a hard task, whereas the more laid back ones had an easier life. Occasionally help is needed from managers or counsellors to explore how to balance the demands of the service and the ability of the worker to meet those demands. Learning time-management skills and how to prioritise tasks is an important aspect of this process.

Family and other role models

Family tradition has a strong influence on career choice, and not just careers in health and social care. Role models are influential at all stages of development, but particularly during adolescence when children are starting to make their own life choices. Usually the most powerful role models will be parents. In Allen's study,[1] 18% of male doctors and 14% of female doctors had at least one medical parent. Other significant figures include grandparents, other relatives or family friends. If any of these role models are in the medical or caring professions, there is a strong likelihood that at least one of the children in the family will follow suit. It may be that people from medical families understand the hard work and commitment required to become a doctor, so are more likely to be successful.

On the negative side, if a child senses that there are disadvantages to being a professional carer, they may be put off and choose a completely different career. A child whose experience is that attention is diverted away from her because the patients' needs are more urgent, or who feels neglected because her parents are working long hours or unsocial shifts, might think that another job would be better.

Sometimes parents have explicit expectations that are conveyed to a child in various ways. Medicine can seem rather like a family business in which succession from parent to child is the norm. It is hard to resist the tradition of several generations of doctors in the family, and this may extend to individual specialties.

Role models also operate at other stages of career progression. When I was offering vocational counselling to junior doctors, I noticed that the choice of surgery as a career specialty was more frequent among women trainees who had worked at a hospital where there was a successful and charismatic female consultant surgeon.

The downside is that if career choices are made to please or appease parents, regret and disappointment may set in later. It is never going to be satisfactory to live out the expectations of other people.

The musician

Stuart is one of four brothers whose parents, both doctors, had emigrated from Eastern Europe in 1939. It was a tremendous struggle for them to overcome prejudice and make a new life in the UK. They were determined that the way for their sons to obtain security and respect was for them to enter the professions of either medicine or the law. Stuart did well at school, but he was more interested in music than in other subjects. He was not allowed to play his instrument at home because of the noise, but he did join the school orchestra.

When exam time came, both his teachers and his parents were shocked at his low marks, and he was made to resit the papers. He still failed to get high enough grades to get into medical school, but he managed to get a place at a school of dentistry, thus satisfying the family honour.

Years later he remained unhappy in his work and at times suffered from depression. When his counsellor asked about his early life history it became clear that he had frustrated ambitions to study music. It was not feasible for him to pursue a full-time course of study, but he did take music lessons and joined a jazz band. He now feels much happier. For him, the final resolution will be achieved when he is able to explain to his parents the emotional cost to him of their ambitions for his career.

Traditions and role models are also often a good influence, pointing to a worthwhile and rewarding career. Paul is an audiologist who is quite clear about what led him into his career with deaf people.[2]

Helping the deaf to hear

Paul always knew that he wanted to be an audiologist. His interest in ears came less from the heart than from the hearth. He had a deaf grandmother: 'She was like a second mum to me. Through her I got used to working with deaf people, and that's what got me into the job.' He has progressed in his career and now works with children instead of the elderly.

Traditions also come from certain schools which have expectations that students will follow a medical career. Some public schools have a 'medical' sixth form for the pupils who are expected to apply to medical schools. Conversely, one junior doctor reported that his prestigious school lost interest in him when it was clear that he was going to apply for a London medical school instead of an Oxford or Cambridge place. It was more important for the school's league-table ranking to have Oxbridge success than pupil success.

Students who are undecided about career choice may be channelled into a path that suits the school or their family rather than their own needs. They may only realise that they are unhappy several years down the line. Long and specialised training makes it difficult for doctors to change track, although this is not impossible. A second career resulting from real personal choice can be enormously liberating. Siobhan was a nurse who decided to change her career.

I wish I had done this before

Siobhan had become a nurse without really considering any other options. Her mother and sisters were nurses. After ten years in the job she became increasingly stressed and recognised that her symptom of backache was a manifestation of this. The relentless pressure of work and expectations to cope with more and more patients in a day-case unit wore her down. She found it hard to say 'no', and always tried to do whatever was asked of her.

When she was off work, incapacitated by back pain, she was forced to stop being busy and had time to think about her situation. She said she had a desire to work in the law, but was diffident about exploring this idea because she thought people would laugh at her. However, her immobility gave her time to find out about qualifications and courses, and eventually she decided to train as a legal executive. Years later she admitted that this was a defining moment for her, and her happiness and success in her new career were self-evident.

The switch from a career in nursing to one in law is interesting, as the legal profession also carries with it respect and the power to influence people's lives.

Family tradition can also influence career choice by the continuation of a childhood role. Imagine a child growing up in a home where illness or disability is familiar. A child in this environment may not realise that her experience is abnormal. She may be comfortable in the presence of illness and naturally gravitate towards a career in one of the caring professions, although dissatisfaction may emerge at a later stage. Steve's story shows how this can happen.

Depression

Steve told me how his mother suffered from depression on and off throughout his childhood. 'If she was on one of her down days I had to get my little brother ready for school and make breakfast for us both. We saw ourselves to school. I used to wonder every day what she would be like when we came home from school. Would there be anything for tea, or would she still be in bed? Now I am grown up with my own kids I still always get the breakfast and take the little ones to school. My job as a family social worker is also a continuation of my childhood role. In my work I often seem to be looking after the children of depressed women.'

Steve began to feel that his choice of work had prevented him from making the transition from childhood to adult life. The pattern laid down early in his life had carried on. When he sought counselling from a careers adviser, he wanted to change his job. But when he understood the process of events, he found that he could apply for a post in a different section that would enable him to change his role and take on managerial (adult) responsibilities.

Continuing in a family tradition is one way of maintaining a familiar environment and a sense of belonging. The significance of belonging is explored later in this chapter in the context of power and influence, and also in relation to the process of self-actualisation.

Social work

Social workers' career choice may certainly be influenced by altruism and family tradition in some cases. For others the injustice of social inequality is the driving force. In the UK, 15% of the population live below the poverty line, defined as 60% of the median disposable income. Social workers are concerned with power, or the lack of it, for their clients. They may be influenced by personal experience of deprivation, and are sometimes driven to work to alleviate for others the problems that they have experienced themselves. My experience indicates that social work is a popular choice for those who have been able to pull themselves out of poverty by gaining educational qualifications. These individuals are well placed to understand the issues and offer a role model for change.

A deprived childhood

Simon had a rocky start in life. His mother, a single parent, found it very difficult to cope. She never had enough money, and she struggled to do a part-time job as well as looking after Simon and his brother. They were often hungry and cold, and they did not have the toys or outings that other children had. Simon felt obliged to start a paid job as soon as he could in order to help the family's finances, and he saw no possibility of going to college or university when he left school. When he later trained as a social worker, his mission was to enable people to have better opportunities in life and not to have to suffer the meagre childhood that he had experienced.

Exclusion, poverty and deprivation cause people to feel disempowered. When social workers help their clients to access resources, this gives them some choice and thereby more control over their lives. A social worker may set out on her career with a mission to redistribute power, but may become disillusioned when this turns out to be more difficult than it at first seemed. Sometimes social workers find that they cannot give clients what they want or need, and in some cases are instrumental in limiting clients' choices. Social workers may be involved in agonising decisions to recommend taking children away from a family. Social workers and doctors are involved in sectioning people under the Mental Health Act, in effect taking away their liberty.

The conflict between care and control is a daily reality. These responsibilities will often feel like very unwelcome powers, adding to the stress of an already difficult job. A desire to help may be thwarted when the reality of a job turns out to be quite different from expectations. Balancing care and control is cited as one of the recurrent stresses of social work.[3] Social workers may find that their wish to do something about poverty and deprivation is at odds with what feels like a punitive and restrictive social policy regime, and may feel that they cannot do a good enough job due to inadequate resources.

A change of career

While she was raising her family, Ann had continued to work in a shop. Once her children became more independent she decided to do what she had always wanted to do, so she applied to train as a social worker. For many years she had taken care of her mother as her health deteriorated, so she had an idea of the kind of needs her clients might have and she felt well equipped to do the job.

She was not prepared for the fact that, when she qualified, her job consisted of assessing people's needs and filling out forms. The clients were then put on a waiting list until funds were available for their care package. There was no time for a friendly chat, to listen or to meet the clients' wider needs for companionship. 'This is not what I thought I would be doing. I feel I am holding out hope and then taking it away again.'

I was not surprised to hear that Ann eventually returned to running a shop, where she did have time to talk to her customers.

Ann was also facing the reality of her own mother's failing health. Part of her disillusionment with the social work profession was a sense of powerlessness to make a difference to her clients' or her mother's lives. All the frustrations that her clients experienced applied to her mother, too.

Those who have never experienced poverty or deprivation may want to help others less fortunate than themselves, but they are in danger of being perceived as superior or moralistic by clients. Caring has a shadow side that may perpetuate a divide that keeps the carer in control. In some cases it shields the carer from having to face her own vulnerability, and the possibility that one day she too may be old or poor or disabled.

Social workers and healthcare workers deal with opposites – health and sickness, wealth and poverty, power and impotence. These are all uncomfortable pairings, because the balance can shift from one side to the other. There is sometimes a sense that by placing oneself firmly in the caring camp it is possible to avoid the negative experiences of illness, poverty or disempowerment. This is a fragile security and it is easily punctured. When career choices have been made in order to preserve a position on the side of the equation that endows health, power or control, it can be devastating when the balance changes.

When a doctor or nurse becomes ill, she may deny her symptoms and try to carry on as though nothing is happening, or at the other extreme she may imagine the worst-case scenario. Social workers who find that they are expected to ration resources instead of giving out help may complain that 'This is not the job I thought I would be doing.' Professional carers often seem to gravitate towards extremes and find it hard to occupy the middle ground. The stress that is provoked by this polarisation is explored in Chapter 4.

The importance of belonging

Throughout the process of growing up, the knowledge and experience that are gained enable a person to become more competent and confident in the world. Sometimes real expertise is inadequate or does not come quickly enough, and an individual may then find other ways of gaining confidence. This may be achieved by joining a group or club that has cachet, or by taking a job with a respected organisation. A sense of belonging helps an individual to feel more confident as she takes on some of the power and protection of the larger organisation.

For some, the prospect of belonging to a profession that carries respect, power and financial reward is an important factor in choosing their career. Working in health and social care may fulfil this need. Medical consultants and general practitioners command great respect and a high salary for the work that they do. Even at the level of low-skilled jobs there is public recognition for those who work in the helping professions. Why do people with jobs that are not necessarily specific to health and social care choose to work in this sector? The esteem that the public has for the whole profession rubs off on the workers in supporting roles as well. It also feels safe to be working in a hospital, a caring environment or a place where people are looked after. This may be one of the hidden psychological reasons for choosing to work in health and social care.

Healthcare: a uniformed profession

The status and security that come from belonging to a particular organisation are reinforced when members of staff wear a uniform. It may be a matter of pride to wear the uniform of a prestigious company or a well-known hospital. Uniforms confer a corporate identity and often include some evidence of rank. They are commonly supplied by the employer, so incur little cost to the worker, although the wearer has no choice with regard to style or quality.

Changes in style have inevitably occurred in response to modern standards. Lace caps and starched aprons are rare nowadays. A new uniform is the scrub suit, with a stethoscope draped around the neck, worn by operating-theatre staff, and familiar from the influence of television shows. This uniform indicates 'I belong to a glamorous profession.' Uniforms also serve a hygienic purpose in that they protect the wearer's own clothes from damage or contamination. In a hospital, by wearing uniform, staff protect patients from infection that might be brought in on street clothes.

Some workers have uniforms that are not issued by their employer, but which are nonetheless recognisable. I recall being told in the 1970s that a social worker could always be recognised by their 'jeans suit.' Social workers are careful not to intimidate their clients and have developed the art of dressing down but not scruffily.

Those who feel constrained by uniform and resent the restriction of ex-pression of their personality through their own choice of clothing will find other ways to demonstrate their individuality, or choose a job that does not require a uniform.

In the case of healthcare, patients may also gain confidence from uniform. From the patient's or client's point of view a uniform tells them to whom they are speaking and that person's place in the hierarchy. For someone who is troubled, confused or sick this may be very comforting.

The power of uniform

An army surgeon returned to normal duties after serving in a conflict zone. After a few weeks he was suddenly overcome with panic and flashbacks of his time in the war zone. He was admitted to an acute psychiatric ward in an NHS hospital where he was diagnosed as having acute post-traumatic stress disorder. With appropriate treatment he recovered and eventually returned to work. However, as sometimes happens in this condition, he suffered a relapse after a few months, and this time he was admitted to a military hospital. He immediately noticed the benefit of seeing the staff in crisp uniform with rank markings and name badges. He felt safe and secure in a familiar environment.

In contrast, the previous ward was friendly and efficient but in a low-key way, and neither doctors nor nurses had any identification other than a name badge. Sometimes it was difficult to tell who was a member of staff and who was a patient. He felt sure that the more secure environment of the military hospital aided his recovery. He knew his place there and he knew what to expect from those who were caring for him.

Uniform also serves a useful purpose in defining the limits of the working day. Putting on a uniform denotes starting work, and marks the transition from personal life to professional life. Taking it off again means finishing work, going home, relaxing and no longer being subject to the stresses of the workplace.

Compulsive caring

Some of the overt reasons for choosing to work in the caring professions also have a subconscious element. Altruism, making restitution for childhood deprivation, following in one's parents' footsteps or wanting the safety of a caring environment are some examples that I have already referred to. Many of the health and social care workers who seek help from counsellors and support services are compulsive carers. They have chosen to work in this sector without necessarily realising that the strength of their subconscious urge to make people better reflects their own needs.

The personality of the compulsive carer, which has been described by Bowlby,[4] is influenced by early life experience. For healthy development it is crucial that a child's infantile needs are met and also that the child learns to be more self-sufficient at the appropriate time as she gains confidence. At birth a baby must be fed, protected from the environment and cared for, otherwise she cannot survive. Little by little she learns to attract attention, to protest when she is hungry, and to reach out and make contact with her environment. Later she can feed herself, move about and relate to those who look after her. Gradually she acquires the skills of self-sufficiency during the process of growing up.

If parents are unable to provide a good enough model of this process by a combination of protection, encouragement and secure boundaries, there may be psychological consequences. It is not always possible to protect children from events such as illness or bereavement. If a parent is physically or mentally ill or preoccupied with other events, they may not respond in a way that enables a child to feel secure. In these situations, a child may start to do things for herself at an inappropriately early age. She may also learn to be helpful and to recognise what to do to help without being asked.

If she unconsciously realises that there is little chance of having her own needs met, she may strive to help others in the hope that eventually things will get better. Instead of being looked after, she becomes a carer, and the roles of parent and child are reversed. If this state of affairs continues, and the child's needs are not met, the repeated cycle of caring in the hope of being cared for becomes a compulsion. This lays the groundwork for a life of looking after other people. The anger and frustration of unmet needs are temporarily buried beneath the impulse to care for others, and it may be many years before they surface again in resentment or work-related stress.

Work is my life

When Kirsty arrived for her first counselling session she was distraught and sat with her head in her hands for some time before she was able to talk about herself: 'I can't go to work because I am not sure if I can adequately respond to my patients' needs.' Her work was home nursing of terminally ill patients. At the same time her son was in hospital awaiting surgery for a serious condition. Her family did not offer any sympathy or support. This made her very angry. Kirsty had some understanding about her vocation to help others, linking it clearly in her mind to her experience as a child. When she was 2 years old her baby brother was very ill in hospital and her mother was preoccupied with the sick child for many months. Kirsty had never had a very close relationship with her mother, and continued to be envious of the special treatment given to the sick child throughout the time she was growing up.

By the time she was 2 years old, Kirsty found that her mother was not there for her. The sick child in hospital got all her mother's attention, and her mother could only turn her attention to Kirsty when the invalid recovered. Kirsty's subconscious wish to make it all better was probably formulated at this point. If the sick child recovered, she might then be able to receive some of her mother's love. Sadly, her mother's attention continued to be diverted to the sickly child, so the subconscious impulse was reinforced. Even as an adult Kirsty cannot get her mother's attention.

Professionally the work that Kirsty does is highly valued and there is much positive feedback from patients and their families. However, in caring for the terminally ill she perpetuates the scenario of unfulfilled hope, as her patients do not get better. She readily admits that work is what keeps her going, and that being forced to stop because she has run out of energy to cope causes her deep distress. She has lost the main source of positive input to her life.

> Counselling enabled Kirsty to receive attention for her emotional needs from an older woman or 'mother figure.' At long last she was able to get the validation she needed, not as a nurse but as a person.

When illness or bereavement occurs in families where there are young children, a child's belief in the ability of her parents to protect her is threatened or destroyed. Klein[5] postulated that a child's response to this may be either to feel a responsibility to restore this power to her parents herself, or to identify with someone who might have this ability. Klein proposed that people often attempt to make reparation for childhood loss or traumas during adult life. In the case of death or illness this restitution might be achieved by taking up a career in healthcare. The Greek myth of Chiron tells of the archetypal wounded healer who compensated for weakness by healing others. The Biblical quotation 'Physician, heal thyself'[6] also refers to the healer as a person in need of help.

Compulsive caring may also arise when encouragement is given in a way that promotes behaviour which is inappropriate for a child's stage of development. For example, if a child finds that caring for others wins approval, she will learn to do this repeatedly. The message is reinforced if approval is not given for other achievements. It may then seem to the child that the only way to win approval and love is by caring for others. It is not necessarily a bad thing to gain approval by caring for others, but it should be balanced by other activities and recognition of other personal qualities.

One result of this early conditioning is a person who often puts other people's needs before their own, but subconsciously expects or hopes for the same in return. The compulsive carer gives to others the care that she would like to receive. She relies on the gratitude of her patients for her own sense of well-being. She may have some insight when she says 'I am always the one people turn to when they are in trouble. I think I am a good listener and I really want to help, but sometimes I just wish someone would listen to me instead.'

Such individuals become dedicated parents, selfless partners and wonderful nurses or care workers. However, the flow of energy into other people's needs can only continue if there is sufficient recompense. Love, approval and respect are the psychological drivers of this behaviour. When this equation does not balance, the carer feels overloaded, stressed and frustrated. The consequences of such overload are explored in Chapter 4.

Compulsive caring takes place at home as well as at work. Here there is another possible source of overload, because if a carer has the same role at work and at home she may not have sufficient emotional energy to maintain both of these. The hoped-for reward of reciprocal caring will be thwarted if she has taken on the caring role for the whole family, because then no one else may know how to do it. A small extra load at home or at work will easily tip the balance from coping into breakdown. Resonance between roles at work and in personal life is explored in Chapter 2.

Fear of death

The loss of a parent or close relative, especially if preceded by illness, may feel so intolerable to a child that a subconscious drive to prevent it happening again induces an impulse to be able to heal, or to prevent death, and so leads them to a career in healthcare. This motivation for choosing a medical career has been investigated by Menninger.[7] Sadly, it may be a source of frustration and despair, as ultimately it is not possible to prevent death.

One consequence of childhood bereavement may be that the remaining parent is too preoccupied or too distressed to give adequate support to the child. Sometimes the child is expected to become a substitute parent. This extra responsibility adds to the emotional burden for the bereaved child.

Bereavement

Hazel and Mike were a successful professional couple. Sadly, Mike developed a rare and aggressive cancer. After treatment he had a short remission, but when the cancer recurred he knew that he would die soon. He and Hazel wanted to prepare their young children for this, so they took care to tell them what was happening in a way that they could understand. On the day when it seemed the end was near, Mike asked for all the family to gather round so that he could say goodbye to them. This was a sad and moving occasion.

The eldest of their three children, now a doctor, recalls this day many years later: 'Dad said to me that I would now be the man of the house and he wanted me to make sure everyone was all right. I know he meant well and it was his way of letting go, but for me it was a terrible burden. I felt I could not break down because the family now depended on me. I was unable to process my own grief. Death still scares me, and I know I avoid terminally ill patients in my work as a GP. I need to address this as it is interfering with my ability to do my job.'

When he attended a training course on loss and bereavement, this GP learned to understand his own grief and to face his patients' deaths with more skill.

Material values

Compulsive caring is one manifestation of disrupted emotional development and the resulting personal vulnerability. Another is the quest for money, power and influence. These status symbols that compensate for powerlessness experienced during childhood may be acquired by choosing a prestigious and well-paid career such as medicine.

There are links between material values and emotional security. Money may become a proxy for love. Parents with demanding jobs and many calls on their time may substitute toys, clothes and trips for quality time with their children. Although a child will welcome these gifts, she will still crave attention, because in reality time is more important than possessions. If this example has been set she may later have difficulty in balancing her work and family life. One trainee doctor said 'I know I chose medicine as a career partly because of the money doctors earn. When I was a child, money seemed important, but I had not bargained for the downside of the long-hours culture. Now I feel it's more important to be able to spend time with my children. They grow up so quickly, their childhood will be over before I have completed my training. I wish I had chosen a different career.'

Income is of course essential, but the pursuit of money at the expense of time with one's partner and children does not lead to happiness. Doctors traditionally can expect to be high earners, but they also expect to work long hours and will admit that family life suffers because of this. Sometimes trainees knowingly accept that hard work and long hours are part of the training process, and endure them in the expectation that rewards will come later.

Emotional detachment

Johnson[8] indicates that emotional detachment and denial of personal vulnerability are common in doctors. These traits are encouraged during professional training, and may help doctors to remain objective when faced with traumatic situations in their work. They constitute a professional defence against loss of control. Professionalism does not seem to allow for the admission of personal weakness.

At the same time, a good 'bedside manner', or the ability to empathise and put patients at ease, is a valued attribute of doctors. Many are able to achieve this, but there is a significant minority who remain inappropriately aloof, distant and emotionally detached from their patients. When emotional detachment spreads into their own personal life, it may lead to marital and relationship breakdown.[9]

The quest for power

For a child to feel secure, her world must be a safe and predictable environment. Traumatic events during childhood result in feelings of vulnerability and powerlessness. According to Klein,[5] children who are affected in this way may develop personality traits that help to restore a sense of security and control. Ritual behaviour, clinging on to a carer and temper tantrums are all ways of trying to be in control. More subtle ways of being in control of others include manipulative behaviour, charm or being 'good.' A child learns what to do to get what she wants, and this is a normal phase of child development. In a healthy family a child gradually learns to feel secure, and controlling behaviour becomes less frequent. For adults, the need to be in control may be manifested in the choice of an influential and well-paid job.

Doctors, nurses and social workers possess specialised knowledge and have the power to change people's lives. Because of their expertise, they are often accorded enormous respect and gratitude. This is a magnificent reward, but it depends on a fickle commodity. If knowledge fails, the power disappears. Individuals with a fragile sense of self-esteem may come to depend on feedback from grateful patients or clients for their ego security and self-validation. Sometimes patients are not grateful, or do not get better. Professional carers often find that they work harder and harder as they chase after these elusive rewards. They may also come to rely on other props, such as alcohol and substance abuse. The difficulty with these solutions is that they only provide fleeting comfort and do not restore low self-esteem. Addiction is explored more fully in Chapter 4.

If power or control becomes the unconscious solution for alleviating emotional inadequacy, it becomes a dangerous tool. When wrongly applied, power becomes a substitute for empathy and care, serving the needs of the worker instead of those of the patient or client.

Abuse of power

Dr Harold Shipman[10] became notorious in 1998 for murdering hundreds of his patients. When he was an adolescent his mother died of cancer, and he is known to have had a history of drug abuse, so it is likely that he experienced some difficult personal conflicts. As he committed suicide while in prison, we shall never know what his inner torments were. What we do know is that he administered fatal injections to his patients. As a doctor he had access to drugs and was trusted to use them safely, but did not do so. He had the power to relieve suffering, but he made wrong judgements as to when to use that power. He may have believed that he was saving his patients from a painful death by allowing them to die under sedation. However, he took upon himself the decision to choose their time of death, going beyond his professional ethics. In the end he chose the time of his own death. The enquiries that followed his case examined the complicity of his colleagues in failing to ask sufficient questions about his professional standards. The respect and trust afforded to doctors allowed Shipman to carry on unchallenged for many years.

Beverley Allitt, a paediatric nurse, was convicted of killing and abusing children in her care.[11] She was found to have deliberately induced illness in her patients by injecting them with insulin or potassium solution, or by partial suffocation. She then heroically 'rescued' them. On some occasions she was rewarded with praise and gratitude, and it is postulated that this was the underlying driving force for her actions. She needed the satisfaction of saving her patients to bolster her own ego. The sicker they were, the more satisfying the rescue was. In her own childhood Beverley had only experienced love and care when she was ill, so love and pain had become confusingly entangled. Her self-esteem depended on illness.

These illustrations show that tragedies can occur when personal vulnerability in carers leads to abuse of power.

Women in the caring professions

More women than men enter the caring professions. Although only a small proportion of nurses are men, they are more likely than women to be in senior positions.[12] Women may choose not to seek promotion to positions of greater responsibility because their primary commitment is to their family. When women take career breaks to look after small children, or decide to work part-time, they fall behind on the career ladder and consequently remain on lower grades with correspondingly low pay scales. Similar career patterns occur in the social work profession. Social work is a mature career choice for some women, and as a consequence fewer years are available for professional development.

Medicine is still a man's world, the language and culture of medicine are male dominated, and the use of sporting and military metaphors and belittling behaviour is common. However, women are catching up. The British Medical Association (BMA) has reported that progressively more women are applying to and being accepted by medical schools.[13] The BMA estimates that women doctors will outnumber men by 2012. Nevertheless, only 25% of the top jobs, namely those of hospital consultants, are held by women. Among surgeons, arguably the most prestigious of all, only 7% are women.[14] Women in Surgical Training (WIST) is an organisation that helps women to progress and to network with other female surgical trainees, and aims to help them to overcome the disadvantages of gender imbalance.

Deliberate policy changes were made in the 1970s when academic excellence was the main criterion for selection of doctors. Clever academics were not always sufficiently empathic to make good doctors, and many became frustrated at the slow pace of change in the NHS. A high level of academic achievement did not necessarily predict success as a doctor. Selection procedures now include markers for empathy and altruism. Factors such as a sense of commitment and previous voluntary work are taken into account. These are perceived to be 'feminine' traits, and may account for the current shift in the gender ratio in medical schools. Unfavourable press reports about the long-hours culture and loss of medical autonomy due to health service reforms are sometimes blamed for discouraging male applicants to medical schools in recent years.

Self-actualisation

Our knowledge of human motivation is based on the observations of Maslow,[15] who described a hierarchy of needs in two groupings – deficiency needs and growth needs. Maslow proposed that basic physiological needs must be met before moving on to the higher levels of safety needs, belonging and esteem. In other words, a person who is hungry can only think about food. Unless she feels safe from predators and protected from the climate, a person will not be able to consider creative self-fulfilment. When her deficiency needs have been satisfied, her self-actualisation or growth needs can be addressed. Maslow points out that the process is always unfinished because, in his opinion, each satisfied need opens the door to another layer of progress.

Alderfer[16] reclassified Maslow's hierarchy into three groups, namely existence, relatedness and growth. He emphasises the specific need of humans to have a sense of belonging. Being part of a family, a community or a working team is important to our sense of self. It is only by interacting with other people, communicating with them and receiving reflected attention that a person can discover who and what they are. By participating in communities, groups or systems we find our place in the world.

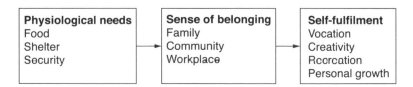

Figure 1.1 The journey to self-fulfilment.

Choice of occupation may be viewed in this context as relevant to more than one human need. An occupation that provides income and security is required to meet basic needs such as those for food and shelter. These needs can be met in a wide range of possible jobs without any high degree of skill necessarily being required.

Occupation may also provide an environment in which an individual can feel a sense of belonging and common purpose, leading to self-esteem. A hospital is a good example of this. Here a worker usually belongs to a team that has a clear purpose. Often a hospital has a strong local identity, perhaps even an imposing building. Everybody knows what it is and what it is for. Being part of a hospital community can endow a worker with purpose and respect.

Once deficiency needs and the need for belonging have been satisfied, the tasks of self-actualisation and personal growth can be addressed. In the complex process of human development, ego ideals are set at an early stage in childhood. Sometimes later modification takes place during adolescence or after traumatic experiences. The drive to live up to these ideals is a major determining factor when considering what occupation to pursue. An unconscious question is being asked: 'Will this job make me into the person I want to be?' In this sense, work is a part of personal identity, and an opportunity to reach towards the achievement of ego satisfaction. For many professional workers the job is fundamental to a sense of self. When early childhood conditioning leads to a need to make reparation for illness, death or deprivation, self-actualisation may be achieved by choosing to work in health or social care. In many cases the task will be successful and psychological healing occurs. The worker gains a sense of satisfaction and patients benefit from their expertise.

Career choice is not the only way to achieve self-actualisation. Family, involvement in the local community, hobbies and voluntary work may all be the source of personal ego satisfaction.

People are often unaware that they are making a psychological choice of career in the expectation of personal fulfilment, so it is not surprising that their dreams are not always realised. The source of the resulting stress, depression or unhappiness may only become apparent when they seek specialised help from counsellors experienced in supporting health and social care workers.

Summary

In this chapter I have explored the conscious and unconscious processes that lead to a career in the caring professions. Altruism, concern for others and a desire to help people are fundamental to care work. These may be taken to extremes when a carer seems to care for patients or clients at the expense of her own and her family's welfare. Altruism can be exploited when more and more is expected from workers who may find it hard to say 'no' when this would cause discomfort to those in their care. The long-hours culture and, for some, protracted training have an adverse effect on family life.

The influence of family impacts on career choice at both conscious and unconscious levels. There may be explicit expectations of certain career choices in some families. This may be in order to maintain family honour, or to continue a familiar emotional and economic environment. Sometimes this is a benign influence, but it may result in decisions that are later regretted. In adult life, career choices can be made on the basis of experience and mature reflection, sometimes resulting in a more satisfying outcome.

Although healthcare workers are concerned with the opposites of health and illness, social workers deal with helplessness and empowerment. Their career motivation may be driven by a desire to alleviate poverty and disadvantage, but often they find that the care they can give is restricted by the need to control scarce resources. Balancing care and control is a recurring source of stress for social workers.

Health and social care is delivered by large organisations offering a wide variety of jobs and careers that attract public recognition and respect. For some workers a sense of prestige, status and authority comes from belonging to an honourable, public and sometimes uniformed organisation. Others gain a sense of safety from working in a caring environment.

Emotional or economic deprivation, illness and bereavement during childhood also influence career choice. Familiarity with illness or death during childhood may lead a child to have a longing for the power to heal, or to make things better, or in some cases to a need to be in control. It sows the seeds of compulsive caring, a syndrome in which the carer is driven by her own psychological needs rather than those of the patient or client.

When emotional or economic deprivation occurs in childhood, psychological protection mechanisms come into play in order to restore a sense of security and control. If these defences continue into adult life, individuals may seek to work in positions of power in order to maintain their personal confidence. Health and social care are examples of occupations that have a powerful impact on life. Health and social care workers with controlling personalities may have excellent technical skills, but are sometimes unable to show the necessary empathy for a caring career. The cases of Shipman and Allitt demonstrate how power can be abused.

Carers have to share their energies between work and family, and they may also act as compulsive carers within the family. Women are more likely than men to be carers both at home and at work.

The final section of this chapter places individual personal development in the context of Maslow's theory of motivation. For the individual, work fulfils several objectives. It helps to provide a roof over one's head, food and economic security. If these needs are satisfied, deeper psychological urges then come into play to satisfy the need for a sense of belonging. At another level, self-actualisation is described as the drive for ego satisfaction, influenced by childhood events, family tradition and other role models. Vocational career choices are made in the arena of unconscious process. We seek out a career that will enable us to achieve personal healing. Some questions are being asked: 'Will this job solve the problems of my childhood? Will it make me into the person I want to be?' Throughout life there are opportunities to attend to the unfinished business of childhood, and working in the caring professions is one way of doing so. For many workers these processes remain in the subconscious. They achieve a balanced and satisfying adult life and work at careers that benefit others without any awareness of their own excessive personal stress.

If the tasks are too overwhelming, or the solutions are unrealistic, or if an unlucky coincidence places extra stress on her personal system, a worker may find that she cannot keep her emotional balance. Managers and staff support services can help to restore this equilibrium.

When health and social care workers seek help for work-related problems, the overt explanation and the presenting symptoms are often only part of the story. It is not surprising that the symptoms are puzzling if the reasons are subconscious. As a counsellor I have learned to look beneath the surface to understand the subconscious motivations that are in operation. Those who provide support can do so more effectively when they understand what the unconscious processes are.

In Chapters 2 and 3 I shall examine the organisational issues for employers and workers in health and social care. The range of problems and symptoms resulting from the interaction of professional carers with the working environment is explored in Chapter 4.

References

1 Allen I (1994) *Doctors and Their Careers: a new generation.* Policy Studies Institute, London.
2 *The Independent* (Careers Section), 28 July 2005.
3 Fineman S (1985) *Social Work Stress and Intervention.* Gower, Aldershot.
4 Bowlby J (1977) The making and breaking of affectional bonds 1. *Br J Psychiatry.* **130:** 201–10; The making and breaking of affectional bonds 2. *Br J Psychiatry.* **130:** 421–31.
5 Klein M (1957) *Love, Hate and Reparation.* Tavistock, London.
6 The Bible. Luke 4: 23.
7 Menninger K (1957) Psychological factors in the choice of medicine as a profession. *Bull Menninger Clin.* **21:** 99–106.
8 Johnson WDK (1991) Predisposition to emotional distress and psychiatric illness amongst doctors: the role of unconscious and experiential factors. *Br J Med Psychol.* **64:** 317–29.
9 Menninger R (2003) Stress: defining the personal equation. *BMJ.* **326:** S107.
10 Smith J (2002) *The Shipman Inquiry: First Report.* The Stationery Office, London.
11 Clothier C (1994) *The Clothier Report.* The Stationery Office, London.
12 Finlayson L and Nazroo J (1998) *Gender Inequalities in Nursing Careers.* Policy Studies Institute, London.
13 British Medical Association Board of Medical Education (2004) *The Demography of Medical Schools.* British Medical Association, London.
14 Department of Health (2004) *Hospital, Public Health Medicine and Community Health Services Medical and Dental Staff in England 1993–2003.* Department of Health, London.
15 Maslow AH (1970) *Motivation and Personality* (2e). Harper and Row, New York.
16 Alderfer C (1972) *Existence, Relatedness and Growth.* Free Press, New York.

Chapter 2

Organisational culture in health and social care

Introduction

In this chapter I propose to explore the importance of organisational factors in health and social care. Management theories about organisational culture are applied to health and social care organisations, and further understanding of these complex and continuously evolving organisations comes from a systemic approach.

Systems theory is a way of looking at how organisations function. It gives insight into the interactions between different parts of organisations such as health and social care. It also shows how workplace systems interconnect with individuals' personal systems in ways that sometimes magnify stress. Equally, systems theory is applicable to the counselling and supervision processes that are involved in staff support services, and can aid the unravelling of difficulties or the modelling of alternative behaviour patterns. Examples from case studies show how systems theory works in practice.

Health and social care is in a process of continuous evolution due to increasing knowledge and technical ability, as well as the changing demands of society. Adaptation to change causes stress for employees. The stages in the process of organisational change are explored in this chapter, and ideas about management of the resulting stress will be considered in Chapter 4.

Next I examine how the individuals who work in health and social care, and the employing organisations come together by means of a contract of employment. There are often subconscious expectations as well as an explicit contract. The motivation for choosing to work in a caring capacity may be influenced by a number of subconscious processes, as described in Chapter 1, and this may result in unrealistic expectations of job satisfaction or psychological reparation. When the culture and ethos of organisations change, workers may find that they are not doing what they thought they were originally employed to do, and it can be difficult to come to terms with this.

Understanding the organisation's culture

Charles Handy is an influential thinker in the study of organisational behaviour. In his book *Understanding Organisations*[1] he suggests that there are four types of organisational culture, and he then uses these to explain the ways in which organisations function. Handy's model applies to health and social care organisations as well as to the commercial world. The four cultures will now be described in the context of health and social care settings.

Power culture is found when a small organisation, or a department of a larger organisation, has a central leader, often a charismatic individual, with other workers reporting to the centre. A section of social services, a hospital department or a board of directors might operate in this way. On a hospital ward the sister in charge sets the tone of the ward. She decides how to delegate the work to the rest of the staff and acts as line manager to the other nurses.

Role culture consists of specialised, often hierarchical departments with defined roles, which report in parallel to a central command or board of directors. Roles are clear, giving security and accountability, but may be stereotyped and inflexible. A hospital would be a typical example. Within the hospital, doctors and nurses, for example, have different training programmes, areas of expertise and line management. Each group exists in a separate role culture. The nursing hierarchy is separate from the medical hierarchy. A ward sister would have no automatic control over the doctors, although they are looking after the same patients. When nurses and doctors communicate with each other the patients benefit. If communication breaks down, it may be difficult to maintain effective care of patients.

Task culture, as its name implies, is project orientated. It consists of groups or teams working on specific issues. The output comes from cooperation between people with a range of skills appropriate to the task in hand. An operating theatre, a hospital ward or a primary care practice might operate in this way. Task culture is potentially flexible and adaptable, but may be more difficult to control than either power culture or role culture. The main focus is the end result.

If the aim is to provide efficient treatment for asthma sufferers in a primary care practice, the team will decide how to do this. It may be that receptionists set up a new clinic and allow self-referral of patients to this clinic. First-line treatment could be provided by nurses with additional training. They might have a set of criteria for referral to the general practitioner on duty or to a hospital emergency department. This system utilises the skills of the patient, the receptionists, the nurses and the doctors. A pre-arranged referral plan helps it all to run smoothly, and each individual trusts the rest of the team to use their judgement appropriately.

The fourth of Handy's categories is the *person culture*. This is less common than the other three, and consists of individuals working more or less independently and perhaps sharing a common philosophy or profession and sharing services. This type of culture has minimal structure and can be difficult to manage. The highly individualistic person culture has always existed in the medical profession, and doctors still cling to the concept of clinical independence. They want to have the freedom to make the best clinical decisions for individual patients, even when this conflicts with the broader needs of the whole community and the economic reality of limited funds.

In the competition for clinical budgets the eloquence of the protagonist and the emotional weight of the specialty often influence decisions, and less interesting bids fall by the wayside. This situation is becoming harder to defend in the face of financial restraint and National Institute for Health and Clinical Excellence (NICE) guidelines. Nevertheless, the personal struggle of doctors who feel that the system prevents them from doing their best for their patients continues to generate anger and disillusionment for some people.

Carroll[2] points out that organisations also have an emotional culture. Individuals bring their personality and their emotions to the workplace. Chapter 1 explored how personality can affect career choice. Health and social care are known as the helping professions, and those who work in this sector perceive that they work in a caring environment, or a *support culture*. This influences both the way they do their job and the way they expect to be treated as employees. Many professional carers consciously or unconsciously expect to be cared for as well as to care for others in their workplace. Workers sometimes have to manage conflicting roles. They may be in a caring environment and have a nurturing role for staff as well as patients, but they may also have to make hard-nosed managerial decisions. If all the staff want to take time off over the Christmas holiday, the manager has to make unpopular and uncomfortable choices in order to keep the department running.

Hawkins and Shohet[3] point out that a *crisis culture* in an organisation may become self-perpetuating. If the staff are constantly reacting to crises, there seems to be no time in which to plan and reflect. Stress levels rise and crises become more likely. In an *addictive organisation*, patterns of behaviour and response tend to encourage dependency and workaholism. These patterns of organisational behaviour are familiar in health and social care, and are resistant to change. However, one of the purposes of this book is to show how an organisation can change and benefit from experience, thus becoming a *learning organisation*.

In his later work, Handy[4] recognised that organisations have evolved and no longer fit so neatly into different types of culture. One result of this evolutionary process is a more flexible organisation consisting of a core management with a series of task forces that report to the centre and outsource many functions. This management philosophy helps modern personal care providers in their aim of continuing to meet the changing requirements of society while at the same time encouraging creativity and open-mindedness. The demands of client-focused and cost-effective services require new ways of working.

There is now more emphasis on teamwork and flexibility between different hierarchies in healthcare. Examples of this can be seen in primary care, where nurses conduct consultations and run clinics for asthma, diabetes and preventive medicine. The introduction of the nurse consultant grade in the National Health Service (NHS) recognises nurses' ability to perform highly specialised roles. Healthcare provision is becoming more flexible, varied and dynamic.

Flexible organisations are often described in terms of systems theory, which is a way of looking at the dynamics of group behaviour. Managers who are providing support for health and social services workers, staff counsellors, human resource managers and others will find it useful to have an understanding of systems theory and the psychodynamics of groups.

Systems theory

Systems in health and social care

Systems theory is a way of understanding how people interact with each other at both an interpersonal and an organisational level. Psychodynamic principles of individual behaviour are also relevant to the collective behaviour of groups. The systemic model consists of interdependent functional units that contribute to make up a whole organism. In a biological model there would be a digestive system, a nervous system and a circulatory system, and so on, forming a complete animal. No single part could survive alone, and all are necessary to the organism's existence.

Organisations consist of one or more interacting parts or systems. What happens in one part has an effect on other parts, and vice versa. Sometimes there is a ripple effect that passes from one part of the organisation to another, and so on, like a chain reaction. Responses also pass back up the line. This might be called a *linear system*. In other cases, the effect causes a feedback response, as in a heating system where the rising room temperature activates a thermostat that leads the control system to cause the boiler to produce less heat. In due course the temperature falls and the thermostat sends a message to switch the boiler back on again, and so on. This is described as a *recursive system*. McCaughan and Palmer[5] explain how systems theory can help managers to understand what happens in organisations.

To illustrate how systems theory can be applied to health and social care, consider a hospital operating theatre. The theatre depends upon the radiology and pathology departments (among others) to provide the information necessary to perform the correct procedures. For example, suppose that a patient with a recurrent cough has an X-ray that shows a shadow on their left lung. When this is investigated, a biopsy indicates that the shadow is due to a malignant growth. The surgeon knows from these test results that she has to remove a tumour from the patient's left lung. Unless she has all the correct information she cannot perform her part of the treatment. The radiology and pathology departments are separate sections, but essential to the work of the theatre.

All of these departments need information technology services, laundry and clerical workers. Within each department there will be leaders and followers, people with specific professional skills, different styles of communication and sometimes disagreements. The operating-theatre manager has the important role of coordinating all the components that are needed for an efficient department. The operating theatre and its interactions with other departments constitute an example of recursive systems. The Chief Executive and the Trust Board members oversee the whole organisation, set the agenda and manage the hospital. With regard to the line management hierarchy the theatre also has linear systems.

Systems may have no explicit ground rules, but nevertheless certain patterns of behaviour will occur and the various individuals assume roles and tasks within those systems. The attributes of systems include the following:

- tasks
- relationships
- communication
- values and beliefs
- knowledge
- complexity.

The above list is not exhaustive, and different systems may have a variety of combinations of attributes.

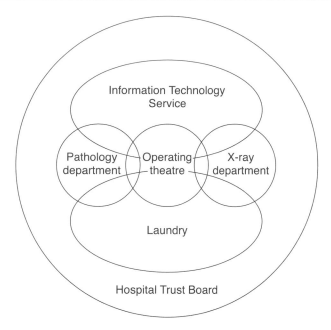

Figure 2.1 Systems in a hospital operating theatre.

Tasks

A systemic group will usually have a purpose – for example, to provide a particular service. Our hospital operating theatre provides suitable rooms, equipment and staff to perform surgical operations. The pathology department provides analytical services for the different hospital departments. One of the tasks of a social service system could be to provide child protection services for the local community. A family constitutes a system whose task may be to create a secure environment for the family members. A social group system may have the purpose of encouraging a particular hobby or entertainment. The operating theatre staff become a social group when they have a departmental night out, and the task here may be to 'bond' or improve relationships within the department.

Relationships

Workers in the operating theatre relate to each other in a command structure of line management. There will probably be several lines of command – nurses, doctors, technicians and cleaning staff all have their own hierarchy of management. They also cooperate by doing their job alongside others with different skills in order to achieve the tasks of the system. They recognise that they form part of a whole and that they need each other in order to achieve the group's purpose. There will often be a power structure consisting of one or more leaders and subordinates. This may be the driving force of the group. However, power potentially creates an imbalance that generates tension and anxiety. Individuals may be in or out of favour, good or bad, and the resulting division or split may hinder the work of the group.

The team members also relate to the patients who are being operated on and who put their trust in the expertise of the whole team. Some workers carry out their job in a dispassionate way, while others make an effort to put patients at ease.

Communication

Members of the group use a variety of means of communication. The theatre manager may put up a list of the day's operations. This informs everyone what work there is to do. Another list may state which members of staff are allocated to each theatre. Within the theatre, verbal communication takes place all the time as the work progresses. Sometimes gestures replace words. Communication with other parts of the hospital could be by telephone or email. Operation notes are written in the patient's case notes, or may be dictated into a tape recorder for later transcription by a secretary.

If messages are unclear, or if some people do not receive the messages, communication will be incomplete. Individuals may be deliberately excluded, either because it is considered that they do not need to know, or as a way of maintaining a hierarchy of power. Communication may be in the form of orders, information, or questions to be answered. You will be able to think of other examples for yourself. Sometimes communication is non-verbal. Body language is a powerful means of communication, but confusion arises when non-verbal and verbal messages are inconsistent. If communication breaks down, the system is unable to carry out its tasks.

Values and beliefs

The values and beliefs of a group come from previous experience. For instance, if the laundry is delayed from time to time, the theatre staff may formulate a belief that the laundry service is inefficient. This may be true, or it may be that the transport service is the culprit. There may be spoken and unspoken rules of behaviour or dress code. For example, 'swearing is not permitted', or 'this is the way we do things in this department.' A newcomer may unwittingly break these rules, but will soon find out when they do so because they then experience their colleagues' disapproval. Disapproval may also be spoken or unspoken. Sometimes a challenge to established tradition results in a change to the group's values.

Knowledge

Over a period of time a group or system builds up a collective knowledge. This is similar in some respects to values and beliefs. Knowledge includes technical matters, the history of the organisation and practical skills. Some of this will be written down, but much of it is carried in the minds of individual members of the group. When this knowledge is shared, explored and developed, the group as a whole benefits. New members of a team are instructed in the department's methods of working. They may bring new ideas with them from previous experience. New techniques and new equipment are regularly incorporated into the system. At the same time as being a functional entity, a system has the capacity to learn and change.

Complexity

Large organisations, departments and social groups usually comprise several interconnected systems. Exchanges within and between systems can be complicated and multilayered. They operate over short-term or continuing timescales. Often other types of organisational behaviour, such as hierarchy and power struggles, will be going on at the same time.

Stacey[6] has written about the complex responsive processes in organisations. Interactions between individuals involve a continuous process of communication. These may consist of words that are spoken, written or electronically transmitted. Non-verbal communication also plays an essential role. Members of groups communicate by means of gesture, posture and expression of emotion. Body language may be a more powerful method of communication than oral language – actions speak louder than words. The dialogue goes back and forth and among the members of a group as they live their life and do their job. This is how ideas are formulated and developed. It is a process that operates at a simple day-to-day level, but also in organisational management and in the complex intellectual arguments of academia. Often these complex interactions take place at a subconscious level. When the system is disturbed the effects become conscious, although it may not be clear how the problem arose until we look at things in more detail.

Systems theory in action

Peter's story is a hypothetical example of systems – his family system and his social work system – interacting in a recursive way.

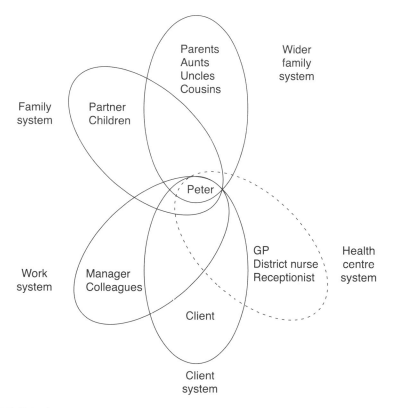

Figure 2.2 Peter's systems.

Peter's systems

Peter is part of a family system together with his partner and their children. Another part of the family is a separate system that interacts from time to time when they get together for birthdays or other events. Peter is also part of a work system. He is a personal carer, one of a team of carers with a team leader and administrative support staff. In the course of his work he goes into the home of a client and becomes part of the client's system. This might involve talking to the client's family members, checking out what needs to be done, or negotiating with yet another system, namely the doctor's surgery. The health centre system is denoted by dots in the diagram to represent occasional short-term interaction. In each of these systems Peter has a range of attributes:

- role
- tasks
- relationships
- communication
- emotions.

These individual attributes are not necessarily fixed. They are similar to the attributes of a system. Some may be shared with a partner, and different roles and attributes will be relevant to home and work. At home Peter's *role* is that of a father. He shares the responsibility for earning money and parenting his children with his partner. He is a good cook, so he produces most of the family meals while his partner spends more time helping the children with their schoolwork. These are their functions or *tasks* in the home. They do not talk much because they have become adept at recognising what needs to be done around the home and they are comfortable with this. They *communicate* non-verbally a lot of the time. Occasionally there are misunderstandings, *emotions* are expressed and they will 'have words' to sort things out.

When he goes to work, Peter is one of several care workers (his *role* at work) and the main responsibility lies with the team leader. His *relationship* with his colleagues is different from his relationship with his family. Carers work mostly as individuals, so there is not much sharing and little *communication* with each other, but Peter has to make sure that he talks to his clients, otherwise he will not know what their needs are. He may have to act as the 'voice' for his client when asking the surgery for medical help. If he is not used to talking much, this might be difficult for him. When there are misunderstandings with his clients, 'having words' may not be the best way to proceed.

Life gets complicated when Peter has to shift from one role to another or adapt his method of communication according to where he is. Some people find this constant balancing act easy. Others are only really comfortable in one particular mode, and try to make it 'fit' the environment in which they happen to be. One way of coping with this would be to find a work system that allows Peter to continue with his preferred role and communication style. Perhaps he would feel more comfortable when he is sufficiently experienced to become a team leader, which would give him more responsibility and a step up in the hierarchy. However, he would probably have to improve his style of communication in order to be successful in this role. Alternatively, he might get a job as a care manager in a residential unit. This might feel like a familiar and comfortable family unit, but would involve working unsocial hours and might detract from his own family life.

All of these processes are probably going on at an unconscious level, and it is only when workers start to feel stressed or out of control that the conflicts between the different systems become apparent. Systems are typically stable and resist pressure to change. A system usually prefers to contain stress within its own boundary. Efficient systems have the capacity to absorb stress and adapt by shifting roles and responsibility according to need. In the above example, Peter might be able to adapt to promotion if his partner is supportive and takes on some of his home tasks while he adjusts to his new role. This might take the form of a negotiation: 'I will cook the tea on Wednesdays so that you can go to a course on management skills. The extra money from the promotion will mean we can all have a better holiday this year.'

A family system that is already under stress may not be able to accommodate an extra load, and the couple's relationship may suffer. If they present themselves to a couple-counselling agency (such as Relate), will the counsellor be able to tease out this systemic tangle? Fortunately, relationship counsellors are used to dealing with family systems, so they may well be able to help the couple to understand why their previously good relationship has gone off balance.

Changes in one system can often have a knock-on effect on another seemingly separate system, due to similar emotions or patterns of behaviour. When things go wrong in more than one system at the same time, especially when the type of problem is similar, rapid disintegration may occur. What might happen if Peter has a row with a client in his care, and is disciplined for this while at the same time he has a row with his father who has asked him to help with looking after his mother? He has been challenged by the person above him in the hierarchy at work, and at the same time he has been challenged by the person 'above' him in the family. He may feel as if his whole world is tumbling about his ears. He cannot face going to work, becomes depressed and is signed off sick by his GP.

Peter is not used to being at home all day, and this saps his confidence even further. Before long he is on a slippery slope to long-term depression, loss of earnings and maybe even redundancy. An intervention to put this in perspective and support him while he deals with these challenges may be all that he needs to stabilise his system. On the other hand, it may be that his family system is vulnerable and some more deep-seated changes may be necessary. Family or couple therapy may enable changes to be made that clarify the roles in the family and improve communication styles.

Layers in the NHS

Another type of system that is commonly seen in health and social care is the layered system. A nurse working on a hospital ward has a role on that ward. The ward is part of the hospital system, which in turn is part of an NHS trust, which is part of the whole NHS. The NHS is a government agency and the Government is chosen by the electorate, which is yet another system. Communication mostly takes place in a linear fashion, consistent with the hierarchical model in this sector.

Suppose the Government decides that, in response to demands from the electorate, certain health targets will be set. This policy is conveyed to the NHS

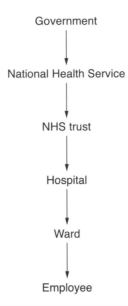

Figure 2.3 Layered systems at work in a hospital setting.

National Executive and on down the chain to a nurse on a hospital ward. She may never have been consulted, and by the time the message gets down to her it may not be recognisable. The message may become distorted as it is passed along the chain, if communication is unclear. The nurse may only perceive that she is expected to work harder, or to fill in an extra form. The correct message will only get through if effective communication takes place at all levels.

When health service reforms required GPs to negotiate contracts for services from hospitals for their patients, the deal was that the money from the contract would 'follow the patient.' Each department would benefit financially from working harder and treating more patients. Hospital staff were asked to fill in forms to identify how many 'patient episodes' had been completed. This was a time-consuming chore, and after a while it became apparent that the forms never left the patients' case notes and the data were never analysed. Staff stopped filling in the forms, and the money did not follow the patient.

This is an example of a reform that failed because the task set by those higher up the chain was unrealistic, and the reasons for the decision were not adequately conveyed to those who had to carry out the task. There was insufficient capacity to process the data. If the chain of communication had included the questions 'Who will process these forms?' and 'What time and equipment will be needed to do it?', things might have been different.

Challenging the systems

Systems are sometimes challenged when emotions become heated. If one person within a department is angry, for instance, the system may have difficulty containing this emotion. A manager who is finding it difficult to meet targets may resent the fact that the targets are unrealistic. She may be short-tempered with a colleague, who then shouts at the receptionist. When a patient calls on the telephone to find out when they can expect to have their operation, the receptionist is unhelpful. The anger is passed around the department and eventually communicated to the patient on the telephone, who is outside the system. This may bounce back when the patient makes a complaint. The whole thing escalates and assumes more momentum. Who knows where it will end? If the manager had been able to negotiate back up the line to set more realistic targets, what would have happened?

Occasionally an employee is referred for help because they are thought to have a personal problem when in reality they are acting out the distress of the whole system. The receptionist described above might be blamed for being rude to a patient. When the patient complains, she might be suspended and referred for counselling or disciplinary action. In reality she was exhibiting the anger that was being passed around the department. This is rather like a problem child who acts out the discord within a dysfunctional family by behaving badly.

The value of systems theory

These examples are necessarily simplified in order to illustrate how systems are involved in organisational function. In fact there will often be many layers and shifting boundaries. The complexity is increased further by the fact that other types of organisational structure coexist with the systems described above. Professional hierarchies are very important in medical systems, and sometimes there may be barriers to communication when doctors only talk to doctors and nurses only talk to nurses. Fortunately, some of these lines of command and control are becoming less restricted, and communication between different management hierarchies takes place more freely now than it did in the past.

Each system has its own rules and homeostatic balance, but cannot exist in isolation. Problems arise for staff when they do not fit comfortably into their system, or the system itself breaks down or fails to communicate with other parts of the organisation. Emotions or processes that occur in one system may be transferred to another system, as in the case of the angry receptionist described above. Alternatively, if there is a similar process going on in more than one system, the worker's normal coping strategies may be overwhelmed. This was Peter's experience when he was disciplined at work and reprimanded by his father.

The systemic approach is extremely useful when dealing with problems that are presented to support agencies and counselling services for health and social care workers. The purpose of these examples is to show that it is possible to understand seemingly dysfunctional processes when they are dissected into their component systems and the attributes of the participants are analysed.

Counsellors may find that what happens in the counselling process replicates or parallels the problem in the workplace or family. When she recognises that this is happening, a counsellor can model different behavioural or coping strategies, and the client may then put these into practice in her own system. This parallel process is a therapeutic tool as well as a way of understanding systemic processes. There are many similarities between systemic workplace counselling and family or couple therapy.

A similar parallel process occurs in the counselling supervision relationship. A supervisor may recognise that what is happening in counselling is repeated in a similar way during supervision. The counsellor and supervisor can then work together to gain a deeper understanding of the client's problems. The supervision process is discussed in more detail in Chapter 5.

Workplace counselling cannot take place in isolation from processes in the employee's personal or home life, as all of the systems may have an impact on each other. The multiple interactions that take place within and between systems are both fascinating and informative – they are a dynamic force for progress and achievement.

Organisational change

How organisational change affects individuals

Over the past 50 years, modern health and social care has been changing at an accelerating rate. There are many reasons for this, but perhaps the most important are new technology, particularly information technology, advances in our understanding of diseases and their treatment, and service users' demands to access the best possible care. Health and social care professionals must take account of cost-effectiveness and evidence-based interventions in the current economic and political climate. Expectations change and the boundaries of what is possible are continually being pushed back. More can be done, so we expect it to be done. Service providers have had to adapt and introduce new ideas in order to meet these new expectations.

Change may have a positive effect when workers gain new skills that enable them to provide treatment more efficiently. However, the emotional impact of repeated change may lead to discomfort, stress and resistance. Ultimately we hope for acceptance, but sometimes exhaustion is the end result. The process of change includes the following stages, although they may not necessarily occur in this order:

- enthusiasm
- fear
- denial
- resistance
- acceptance
- exhaustion.

Enthusiasm

The immediate response may be that change equals stress, but not necessarily negative stress. Some people thrive on change. It is a learning process that can bring excitement, variety and new opportunities. Someone who accepts that change is inevitable and is proactive in the process can perhaps influence how the change is carried out and possibly take her pick of the benefits.

Fear

Employees are expected to be adaptable in implementing change, but modernisation also threatens job security. A worker may perceive that she no longer fits her employer's requirements when new job descriptions replace familiar ones. She may fear that she will be unable to adapt to new practices. Sometimes job losses are inevitable. There may be a greater chance of success when managers try to engage the goodwill of their colleagues and harness their cooperation and enthusiasm in finding new solutions and setting and evaluating targets.

Denial

Another reaction may be to dig in, refuse to accept the change and carry on as though nothing has happened. Eventually this strategy fails because the change usually happens anyway. A person with her head in the sand may then have little choice about the consequences. She may be obliged to accept the reforms, but remains disgruntled and dissatisfied. Often she will take the opportunity to leave the organisation either by choice or by redundancy.

Resistance

Organisational change in the NHS aims to make the system more flexible and responsive to change, although at times reforms have failed due to resistance from staff, as in the NHS reforms of the 1970s. Gradual change carries the danger that it might be imperceptible and ineffective. Consultation with the front-line staff and the clients will often generate useful insights and new ideas, but may also produce the response 'It will never work.' Another danger of consultation is that in the end changes may be imposed despite the views of those consulted. This can cause a very negative backlash. If senior managers try to make reforms and the workforce is not consulted, the people who have to implement the changes may not have faith in the new way of doing things. When reorganisation fails, the response is often to reimpose control, especially financial control. This is perceived as yet more change. Confusion and chaos may follow, and staff morale and effectiveness suffer.

Acceptance

There is no going back from the advancement of knowledge, and workers generally realise this, so they accept that change is a fact of life. They loyally comply with new practices and carry on working. This may mean working differently, and it often means working harder.

Exhaustion

Sometimes change results in an increase in workload that takes place gradually over a period of years and remains unnoticed until, in response to a seemingly trivial event, breaking point is reached. Alternatively, repeated cycles of change may occur until staff eventually lose their resilience and can no longer keep going, so they become exhausted. The effect is often that one person becomes the symptom carrier for the system, is no longer able to cope and is forced to take time off work.

Ruby in overload

Ruby has been a receptionist for 15 years. In the beginning her job was to prepare lists for clinics, make appointments and welcome patients to the department. Over the years the number of consultants in the department has increased from two to four, doubling the number of clinics. A much wider range of technical procedures is performed in the department, by many more technicians. Some procedures that would have previously required admission to hospital are now carried out on outpatients. All of these require appointments, telephone calls and case notes.

The remit of Ruby's job widened enormously, and the number of patients she had to deal with increased accordingly. All the while Ruby cheerfully carried on coping. She benefited from computerisation and more efficient methods of working, but there was no escaping the fact that she had to work much harder than before. In addition, she is such a helpful and friendly person that all the staff used her office as a place to congregate and chat. They asked her to do a variety of administrative tasks that they could arguably do themselves. Having her office used as the gossip station made her working environment noisy and overcrowded.

Finally she reached a point where she felt that she just could not cope any longer. She was unable to face going to work, was signed off sick by her doctor with a diagnosis of stress, and remained off work for seven weeks.

This gave her a lot of time in which to think. Ruby realised that perhaps she had become too helpful and that this had added to her legitimate workload. As a result she resolved to make some changes on her return to work. She now keeps a book of requests and anyone who wants her to do something extra must write it down. Often it is easier for them to do it themselves than to write it down. Also they can see how many other jobs are on the list. Unnecessary chatter is banned, and Ruby asks people to go away if they are getting in her way!

At the same time her manager had realised that Ruby's office had become chaotic, and while she was away steps had been taken to tidy up piles of case notes. A new chair had been ordered, as Ruby is quite short and her old chair was unsuitable for her. An assistant has been brought in from the secretarial bank to help, and each morning there is a staff meeting so that everyone has an opportunity to share any concerns they may have.

In the above example the problem has therefore been addressed from two angles – that of the individual and that of the administration. Both eventually realised that change had overtaken them and that some adjustments were needed. Unfortunately, Ruby had to reach a state of exhaustion before this was recognised.

The impact of organisational change

It may seem ideal for change to be implemented gradually and after consultation with those who will be enacting the new practices. However, external factors dictating change may mean that this ideal is not possible. Changes in Government policy, treatment for new diseases or responses to economic constraints may all have to be introduced rapidly.

Organisational change always has an impact on employees, and is frequently cited as a major cause of increased stress. Necessary change brings anxiety and resistance that affect staff morale even when there will ultimately be benefit.

When organisations and individuals are working close to their limits of capability, the additional stress of change may cause overload and breakdown.

In some cases, change involves taking on a new role. This may be part of planned career development, or it may be imposed by reorganisation. Transition is helped by rites of passage, such as graduation ceremonies, leaving parties and changes of workplace. Sometimes the new role will have visible signs of promotion, such as a bigger office, a personal assistant, a better computer or a larger number of staff. However, leaving a role involves giving up some familiar tasks and this may be surprisingly hard to do. The comfort factor of work that is within one's competence zone is very powerful. When a person takes on a new role without giving up her old one she experiences stress. The apprenticeship system of medical training is particularly prone to this problem because promotion is often within the same hospital or even the same department. Moving on to learn new skills while teaching someone else to do one's old job is frustrating. How much easier it is to do the job oneself than to watch a new trainee make a mess of it. Learning the art of delegation is part of the process of career advancement.

Another aspect of role overload involves the taking on of additional roles in another part of the employee's life. The joy of becoming a parent brings extra responsibility. The death or illness of a relative entails spending time on other family business. These have a knock-on effect which means that there is less energy available for work. Priorities have to be reassessed to take account of such life-stage milestones, and work may get a smaller share of the pie, at least for the time being. The effect of extra responsibility is magnified if it resonates with what is happening in other systems, as described above in Peter's story.

When change is expected, uncertainty about what the impact will be is in itself stressful. Just as with serious illness, waiting for the diagnosis is worse than coping with bad news. Staff support services can help by being aware of what is going on in the wider management of the organisations that they serve, and encouraging open communication. They may be involved in consultation processes in anticipation of change, and can support staff who are experiencing difficulty in coping with change.

Contracts

Spoken and unspoken expectations

The NHS and social services exist to meet the needs of the population for good healthcare and social security. They are public organisations under Government control. Workers have contracts to do specific jobs with specified conditions and rates of pay. The requirements of the organisation and the expectations of the worker are brought together in the contract of employment. Contracts are seldom as clear-cut as they seem, and people working in different parts of the same organisation will sometimes have different contracts (e.g. if some services are contracted out to other companies). If a contract is not perceived in the same way by both parties, conflict or even litigation will result.

The measurable reward for work is money, and this must be equitable and fair by comparison with that for others working for the same organisation. Generous pay awards to senior managers when pay for workers lower down the scale is being squeezed cause outrage. For professional carers the intangible rewards of self-fulfilment and improving the lives of their patients or clients may be at least as important as the financial return, but are rarely mentioned in job descriptions or discussed at interviews.

Contracts do not usually refer to the psychological rewards or disadvantages of a post. We have already seen in Chapter 1 that there are many possible hidden agendas for health and social care workers, whereas by and large the employing organisation has a clear idea of what it requires. Subconscious motivation for workers in health and social care has an important bearing on the contracting process. What they want from their job may not be the same as what the employer is offering, and neither party may realise this.

A job description may ask for qualities such as commitment and specific skills. Sometimes job satisfaction or intellectual challenge is offered. The employer may also expect adaptability, moral integrity, loyalty and the ability to work as a member of a team. It may sometimes seem as if workers are expected to achieve the impossible. Will the organisation offer loyalty and commitment in return? If the employer is an 'Investor in People', what does this imply? The unspoken message is that they care about their employees and want to encourage their personal development, but will they actually do this? In the past perhaps it was realistic to expect that the NHS would offer loyalty and commitment (job security) to its employees, but now the pace of change means that this is no longer always the case.

Existing employees may find that changes in the delivery of health and social care result in restructuring of departments, leading to redundancies and changes in the type and mix of staff required. Many surgical procedures can now be performed as day cases, and wards have been adapted to make this type of working possible. Modern communication systems have removed the need for a rank of telephone operators to connect callers to departments. Fewer secretaries are needed when letters and reports are transmitted electronically, or at least the duties expected of a secretary are different. Sometimes workers are forced to reapply for jobs with updated terms and conditions. The subconscious 'deal' described by Jarvis[7] is not what it used to be. Employees' expectations lag behind the pace of change of organisational management, resulting in a mismatch in subconscious expectations. As a result, workers may become disillusioned and feel that they are not doing the job they originally set out to do.

Public service organisations also have an implied contract with the users of the service that will have been laid down by the Government or the local authority. Difficulties arise when the expectations of users do not match what is being provided. Staff may have a personal standard of care that is higher than can be achieved within the budget, or their standard may relate to a different agenda (as in the case of social workers like Ann, described in Chapter 1, who want to help people rather than ration resources).

Problems also occur when receivers of care do not respond in the expected way.

A fun day out

Ellie is an events coordinator for a young people's housing project. She organises events to encourage the clients to develop social skills. Having asked around for ideas about what her clients would enjoy, she booked an outing to a theme park. She made a list of those who would definitely take part. A coach was booked and everyone was informed of the meeting place and time. In the event, hardly any of the participants turned up. The reasons given were 'overslept', 'couldn't be bothered' or 'didn't feel like it.' Ellie was bitterly disappointed by their lack of interest, and felt personally responsible for the failure of the event. Her manager was concerned that the charity funding the event would feel that their funds had not been wisely used, and that future funding might be put at risk.

Ellie's view of the subconscious contract was 'I will organise a fun event, and if you have agreed to participate you will actually do so.' From the clients' point of view the subconscious expectation was that 'I can go if I feel like it' or 'It might not happen.' These clients may have had little experience of reliable arrangements, and in their world there might be no certainty that the event would happen. In the past they may have been disappointed so many times by failed outings that they would have no confidence that this trip would actually take place.

Carers working with vulnerable people have to accept that their clients may not always be able to appreciate what is being provided and may waste resources through lack of confidence in the system. This can be disheartening for carers even when they have an understanding of the difficulties posed by clients' previous negative experiences.

In the above example there is a triangle of contracts in which each participant interacts with two other agents, as shown in Figure 2.4.

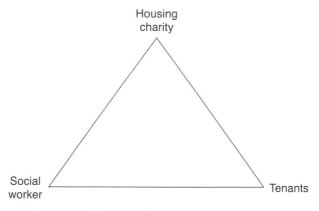

Figure 2.4 Contracts between a housing charity, its tenants and a social worker.

In this case the housing charity sets out to provide a service to tenants, and to do this it employs a social worker who is paid by the charity and organises events for the tenants. The tenants use the services provided by the charity and the social worker. A contract of employment usually defines the role that the worker has in the organisation, in this case to provide social activities for the tenants.

The contract between the housing association and the tenant is clear. In exchange for a home, the tenant pays an agreed rent and abides by rules set down by the landlord. However, the contract between the social worker and the tenants is not clear. We do not even know whether the tenants want to have activities organised for them.

If expectations do not match reality or if the organisational ethics do not match the worker's personal ethics, role incompatibility may occur. For example, a social worker who sees herself as a saviour will be unhappy if her job involves restricting the distribution of scarce resources. We may question whether the contract is between the employee and the employer or between the employee and her professional or personal ideals. A consultant may be more interested in the potential for a job to provide opportunities to pursue research in a chosen specialty than in the waiting list for routine operations.

Thus there is a complex interaction between the worker, the employer and the user of the service. At yet another level the Government has a contract with service providers and also with the electorate, who are ultimately the service users. There is therefore plenty of potential for mismatch of expectations and for conflict between the various conscious and unconscious roles that the worker is trying to fulfil. If the worker's psychological needs are not met or there is role conflict, stress will occur, and in many cases this is what prompts workers to ask for help.

Contracts in workplace counselling

When an employee seeks help from a workplace counsellor, a different set of contractual relationships exists. This becomes more complicated when we also include a supervisor in the overall picture.

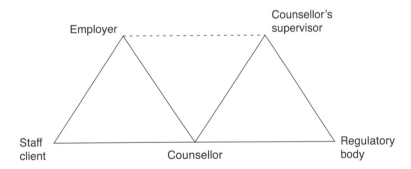

Figure 2.5 Contracts in workplace counselling.

Figure 2.5 shows how the counsellor maintains a professional relationship with four different bodies. She is employed by the organisation to provide counselling for staff clients. She reports to a counselling supervisor, and she must also be a member of a professional regulatory body that lays down standards of practice. Regular supervision is a professional requirement for maintaining her registration. In some cases her supervisor is also an employee of the same organisation. In a situation of this complexity, conflicts of interest are likely to occur. For example, under what circumstances should the counsellor disclose information about the client (staff member) to the employing organisation?

Although a counsellor is primarily concerned with the welfare of her client, she cannot ignore the fact that she also has a responsibility to the employer. Confidentiality is rarely absolute, and this must be explained to the client. Confidentiality may have to be breached if criminal activity is disclosed, or if the safety of the client or another person is at risk. A counsellor who decides to step outside the boundary of confidentiality will usually try to discuss this with her client and if possible seek her agreement. She may need the support of her supervisor and her professional body in this situation. Jenkins has explored the ethical and legal aspects of counselling contracts.[8] Professional conduct is increasingly the subject of litigation, so counsellors must remain aware of their legal duty to clients and employers.

Similar dilemmas about confidentiality may apply to the counsellor–supervisor relationship. For example, if the supervisor decides that a counsellor is not fit to practise, for health or other reasons, she must if possible explore this with the counsellor and decide upon a course of action in accordance with ethical good practice. Counselling supervision is a helpful forum for exploring the systemic aspects of workplace counselling (*see also* Chapter 5).

Summary

I have considered the management of health and social care in terms of organisational culture. Power culture involves individuals or teams reporting to a central leader. Role culture often consists of parallel hierarchies with defined roles, and there may be little communication between the separate strands. Task culture has a flat structure with a specific outcome as its main focus. When charismatic individuals work more or less independently this is described as a person culture. All of these cultures exist in health and social care. I have also considered the concept of emotional culture in organisations. In the context of health and social care, support culture, crisis culture and addictive culture are frequently encountered. Health and social care – the helping professions – are assumed to be caring organisations, and employees expect to be cared for as well as being the providers of care.

Further understanding of organisations comes from adopting a systemic approach to examine the interactions of groups, teams or departments. Work-place systems also impact on personal and social systems. Systemic cooperation is important for efficient working. Systems are also subject to complex psychological processes. Case histories illustrate systemic synergy and parallel process. Understanding the dynamics of systems helps managers and counsellors to resolve problems and to change dysfunctional practices.

Health and social care is in a process of continuing development. Change is brought about simultaneously by technological progress and the establishment's strategies to meet increasing expectations of service users. Individual workers respond to the process of change in a variety of ways. They may be willing to adapt and be enthusiastic about changes that promise to improve outcomes or make their work more efficient. Sometimes they are reluctant to change, or when they do accept the need for change, they become disillusioned when the predicted benefits do not materialise. The additional stress resulting from changing practices may cause overload, exhaustion and breakdown for individuals and organisations. Managers and counsellors will find it useful to understand these processes when they are helping staff to cope with implementation of change in their organisations.

Organisational change has another effect in that it may result in changes to the contract between employee and employer. There is often an implied or unspoken contract as well as the explicit contract. When this unspoken contract is broken or not fulfilled, workers become disappointed and angry. Tension also arises from the unspoken needs of those workers who perhaps unconsciously expect gratitude, respect and psychological reparation when these are not always possible. Managers and counsellors working for staff support services will sometimes find that the process of helping stressed workers involves clarifying what the 'deal' really is. A counsellor must remain aware of the contract that she has with the employer as well as with her client.

Chapter 3 examines the impact of organisational issues on different groups involved in the delivery of health and social care services.

References

1   Handy C (1993) *Understanding Organisations* (4e). Penguin, Harmondsworth.
2   Carroll M (1996) *Workplace Counselling.* Sage, London.
3   Hawkins P and Shohet R (2000) *Supervision in the Helping Professions.* Open University Press, Buckingham.
4   Handy C (1996) *Beyond Certainty.* Arrow, London.
5   McCaughan N and Palmer B (1994) *Systems Thinking for Harassed Managers.* Karnac, London.
6   Stacey RD (2001) *Complex Responsive Processes in Organisations.* Routledge, London.
7   Jarvis CA (2004) *Changing the deal.* PhD thesis, University of the West of England, Bristol.
8   Jenkins P (2006) Supervising workplace counsellors: accountability and duty of care. *Counsel Work.* **51**: 8–10.

The impact of organisational culture on those working in health and social care

Introduction

In Chapter 2 the theoretical aspects of an organisation's culture were considered in the context of health and social care. This chapter explores the impact of organisational culture on the individuals who work in health and social care.

Examination of the evolution of the National Health Service (NHS) shows how repeated cycles of change and a significant cultural shift have taken place. When it was set up, the NHS arguably created false expectations of universal provision of free healthcare. There is now an explicit requirement to deliver best practice in a cost-effective way. Major changes have also occurred in the training and professional status of nurses. Doctors and other professionals have had to contend with the increasing pace of change in medical knowledge and a more sophisticated and demanding clientele.

Stress may be caused by specific factors operating in different sectors of the caring professions. I shall explore possible sources of stress in private medical care, complementary medicine and care in the community.

Historically, social welfare has undergone profound changes that are similar to those seen in healthcare. The social work profession has gained a coherent identity to undertake the difficult task of alleviating poverty, exclusion and deprivation. I shall explore the impact of dealing with ambivalence about the issues of care and control, and refer to the prevalence of a blame culture that may cause problems for social workers. Systemic interactions, parallel process and projection are shown to be particularly relevant for social workers. It is important for managers and social workers to understand how they may become drawn into psychological processes such as the drama triangle, and to make sure that relevant support and supervision are provided.

The development of professional regulatory bodies will be explored. These organisations began as protective groups to maintain the interests of a select membership, but are now important for upholding professional standards of competence that protect patients and clients from harm. They may be involved in the investigation of complaints of professional negligence. The impact of such investigations on individuals can be severe. I shall also consider the damaging effects of bullying, and the importance of anti-discrimination measures.

Finally, there is a section on staff benefits. Despite all the changes, and the stress of dealing with difficult problems and psychological pitfalls, there are many benefits for health and social care professionals.

Understanding the NHS today

Clues from the past

Expectations of healthcare for the whole nation were dramatically altered in the post-war years. The Beveridge Report[1] set out proposals for a comprehensive social insurance system in 1942. In 1948 the NHS was introduced by the then Health Minister Aneurin Bevan. The principle that everyone should receive the healthcare they need without cost at the point of use, regardless of income, was a noble one. For the first time the State would care for everyone 'from the cradle to the grave.' In principle a healthy population would cost less. Preventive medicine would be less expensive than remedial treatment. In practice, of course, this was a fallacy and Bevan himself recognised this. Expectations rose. People who were cured of infections such as tuberculosis lived on to develop other conditions. With advancing medical knowledge, conditions that had previously been incurable became treatable and hitherto undreamed of interventions are now possible, such as joint replacements, chemotherapy and gene therapy, to name just a few. Treatment also leads to iatrogenic diseases due to the adverse effects of drugs. For example, suppression of the immune system by chemotherapy results in septicaemia, and the use of broad-spectrum antibiotics leads to infection by antibiotic-resistant bacteria.

The NHS started to run out of money in its early days, and gradually charges were introduced for some specific services such as prescriptions, dental treatment and spectacles. The expectation of free and universal treatment lives on, but this is not realistic. The idealistic message was just what people wanted to hear, and this is the message that is remembered even though it has not been true for many years. Responsibility for health was transferred from the individual to the Government. Instead of looking after their own health, people feel entitled to be looked after. More and more treatment is provided, but people feel less healthy. This irony was explored by Ivan Illich in his book *Medical Nemesis*.[2]

Counsellors, managers and human resource professionals are familiar with the idea that healthcare workers would also like to believe in free universal care. They are both receivers and givers of care. I often hear nurses or social workers say that restrictions on time and resources do not allow them to give the standard of care that they would like their own loved ones to receive. They are applying a private standard to a public service. Unfortunately, the two cannot be the same. We need public services because it is not possible to provide the solutions ourselves on an individual basis. For example, it is very hard to admit to being unable to provide 24-hour care for a parent who is suffering from dementia. It is more than one person can do, however noble their intentions. The pain of this sense of inadequacy may turn into anger that can be inappropriately directed at the agency that provides the care, or into self-blame. Nursing and personal care are so closely linked to the way family members look after each other that the boundaries between professional care and family care for loved ones are indistinct. Healthcare workers often feel that they are caught between their personal commitment to patient care and the financial and managerial restraints placed upon them by the organisation. The result is a stressful conflict of roles. The gap between ideal and reality causes much frustration and unhappiness. The task for managers, human resource professionals and counsellors in health and social care includes helping staff to work with that discrepancy and providing support when it becomes difficult to cope.

NHS hospitals

The crisis in healthcare in the 1970s led to an explicit strategy to change the culture of the NHS. In 1983 the Griffiths Report[3] called for changes in the hierarchical line management system, but the reforms failed due to internal resistance to change and economic restrictions. There was an increase in financial controls and privatisation of hospital services such as cleaning and catering. As a result, managers are now responsible for departmental targets and budgets.

In-house training and development programmes are available for recruits to NHS management. At the bottom of the hierarchy, staff with minimal qualifications are employed in basic jobs but can expect to be given training opportunities to advance themselves. There is a tradition in the NHS of internal promotion that enables people to progress to positions of responsibility. In this way late developers and those wishing to change career are provided with excellent opportunities. The danger is that training is sometimes inadequate and change is implemented too rapidly, resulting in insecure managers who cannot manage their staff properly. Both managers and staff are harmed by this and present themselves for help with the resulting feelings of stress and inadequacy. Low morale spreads to the whole department if it is not rectified.

At the other end of the scale, management expertise is sometimes injected from other industries when senior appointments are made. This recognises the potentially stifling effect of closed systems and is a welcome modernisation. Even so, existing staff may feel insecure when outsiders are appointed and the stability of the system is threatened.

Working for Patients,[4] a Government White Paper, introduced reforms that took place in 1991, leading to decentralised management, a purchaser–provider split and a client-orientated culture. Healthcare is now delivered by NHS trusts. Progressive improvements mean that the concept of what constitutes good health is continually advancing. The criteria for healthcare have changed. *The Health of the Nation,*[5] published by the Department of Health in 1992, provided a strategic approach to the overall health of the nation by focusing on five key health issues. *The Patients' Charter*[6] sets out patients' rights and the standards that they can expect from the NHS. In addition, new initiatives are being pushed forward by the NHS Institute for Innovation and Improvement[7] to optimise staff development, flexibility and retention.

The modern commitment of the NHS is still to deliver both quality and quantity of care to the population. We can monitor the changes and find out whether the objectives are being achieved by analysing the vast amount of information that is available. Collecting statistics is another task that has been added to the list of jobs for health and social care professionals. Many resent this, as it takes up time that they would prefer to spend on face-to-face treatment.

Training and organisation of the nursing profession have been undergoing changes that reflect changes in other parts of the NHS. Historically, nurses were employed to work on hospital wards and training took place in a school of nursing within the hospital setting. Most of their learning would have been on the job, in direct contact with patients. They learned by observing and working with more experienced colleagues, interspersed with regular blocks of classroom teaching. At the end of this training they became state-registered nurses (SRN) or, later, registered general nurses (RGN). If a nurse wanted to do so she could go on to specialise – for example, as a midwife or community nurse – or progress up the hierarchy in hospital.

In the 1990s there was a move to raise the professional status of nursing. Many nurses felt undervalued and also felt that their work was subordinate to that of doctors. From 2000, changes to nurse training have had a profound effect on the whole profession, as was the intention. Trainees now undertake a university degree or a diploma course and receive an academic training, with placements on hospital wards for practical work experience. This reversal of the priorities acknowledges that nurses have the ability to study and understand their work in greater depth. It is empowering and a boost to confidence. Nurses are also able to take on managerial responsibilities that expand their career potential and build bridges across the traditional hierarchical structure of the NHS. Some choose to study for postgraduate qualifications such as the MBA to further increase their skills.

Inevitably there was a gap in the provision of bedside nursing care when these changes took place. A new grade of healthcare assistant was created to ensure continuity of care. Routine tasks on the wards are carried out by those with training in practical skills as opposed to intellectual or managerial skills. Registered nurses undertake specialist care, planning and managerial roles. These changes have not been comfortable. Some do not like the distancing of nurses from bedside care, as this conflicts with the image we used to have of nurses ministering to the sick. Role conflict and coping with change are recurring themes for stressed staff.

Modern management of NHS hospitals has also had a profound effect on doctors. The previous hierarchical way of running hospitals suited the exclusivity of the medical profession. It kept power in the hands of the consultants. Decentralisation, increasing financial controls and patient-focused targets have diluted this power. Many doctors have taken the opportunity to gain management skills and to engage with the modern philosophy of the NHS. However, if a doctor is reluctant to let go of her clinical practice, she shoulders an extra workload of management while continuing to work face to face with patients. Combining a management role with clinical care means trying to do two jobs at once, so it is not surprising that stress levels are high. Doctors in the training grades now look at consultants – their career role models – and no longer envy their achievements. The peak of the profession is less appealing than it used to be.

Well-informed patients who research their own disease sometimes question the treatment they are offered. Doctors no longer have exclusive access to medical information, and may find that gaps in their knowledge are exposed. The superiority of the profession is threatened. Encouragement of patient responsibility and a client-led health service have raised expectations, so that patients are no longer willing to accept what they are offered without question. They will not tolerate mishaps or second-rate treatment. As a result, more doctors and other health professionals are facing the stress of complaints and litigation. Managers also face scrutiny if the problems are traced back to policy decisions or inadequate supervision. Ultimately patient care should improve, but the effects of these additional sources of stress can be overwhelming for staff. The symptoms and management of stress are explored in more detail in Chapter 4.

Recent regulations with regard to working hours provide junior doctors with some protection from the stress of overwork. Sometimes the effect of these rules is to force doctors to squeeze more work into a shorter time. Doctors who are eager to improve their skills and make professional progress are concerned that shorter working hours give them fewer opportunities to gain experience. It may be good for their work–life balance, but it is bad for professional achievement. Balancing work and personal life is one of the perpetual struggles for doctors, and a frequent cause of stress when it seems that unacceptable compromises have to be made.

Primary care

Present-day primary care has moved a long way from the single-handed general practitioner who did everything for the patients in the community. Delivering babies, treating and advising on the whole range of illnesses, performing minor surgery, making up medicines and calming the mentally ill all fell within the remit of the general practitioner. A GP would also often be a pillar of the community. The health needs of the community are now very different, and this is reflected in the way in which care is delivered.

Primary care has evolved in a way that now includes a range of other professionals in a team-based structure. It is less hierarchical than the hospital system. Every member of the team is valued for their particular contribution. Here the predominant stresses are perhaps more concerned with the relentless increase in the expectations of service users and the political pressure to meet those needs. Many GPs willingly engaged with modernisation, introducing computerised record keeping and working with the primary care trusts when they were set up. However, some now feel overwhelmed by bureaucracy and exhausted by repeated cycles of change. GPs would prefer to spend more time with patients instead of filling in forms and attending meetings.

Despite working with a range of colleagues, GPs can feel extremely isolated. In individual consultations with patients a GP may face a succession of life-or-death decisions without access to the immediate support that is available to their hospital colleagues. These responsibilities weigh heavily and add to the stress of the high workload and the need to keep up with advances in knowledge. Caplan[8] noted that depression and suicidal thinking are prevalent among doctors working in general practice. Brewin and Firth-Cozens[9] have reported that the traits of perfectionism and self-blame when things go wrong are significant stressors for some GPs.

Primary care is the buffer zone between the healthy population and specialist medical treatment. GPs often feel that they are the gatekeepers to hospital care, and this can be a very uncomfortable position. They may have to face the anger of patients who cannot get what they want. GPs are often expected to determine fitness for work and eligibility for social security benefits. Health needs and welfare needs are intimately interlinked, making primary care an interface with care in the community and the work of social services.

Private medical care

Opting for private medical care is a personal choice for some, when prompt treatment and a say in the selection of medical practitioner are a priority. Companies that offer private medical care to staff as a fringe benefit have an eye to the fact that cutting out delays in treatment means that workers are likely to be off work for a shorter period of time. Where there are long waiting times for surgery, people who would never previously have considered private healthcare are now choosing to pay rather than wait months or years for treatment. In some cases NHS trusts purchase private treatment to fulfil their obligations to meet waiting-list targets.

Stress issues for staff working in the private sector reflect this diversity of patients. Workers occasionally harbour resentment of demanding patients who naturally feel that if they are paying over the odds they should receive a better standard of service. They may sometimes feel more like hotel staff than hospital workers. Cost is an issue in private medicine, too, and staff may find that financial restraints are even greater than in the public sector. Nurses and doctors may move from the public to the private sector, and sometimes work for both at the same time.

There has long been concern about the boundaries between NHS and private healthcare. Staff members are angered when they feel that resources intended for NHS patients are being siphoned off into the private sector. Services such as pathology, pharmacy and radiology are particularly vulnerable to this. Increased openness will encourage staff to speak out if they suspect malpractice, but they may need support in doing so. Another boundary issue is that members of staff who work concurrently in both sectors may take their problem behaviour with them. For example, when I was providing counselling to different members of the operating-theatre staff in a private hospital and in an NHS hospital nearby, I realised that the underlying problem was the domineering behaviour of the same surgeon who worked in both locations.

Complementary medicine

Complementary medicine has expanded in response to patients' dissatisfaction with conventional medicine. This also reflects the wish of many patients to take responsibility for their own health, both by preventing illness and by choosing treatment such as osteopathy, homeopathy and herbal medicine that may not be available on the NHS.

Many of the issues relating to compulsive caring, rescuing and coping with insoluble problems are relevant to complementary practitioners. A chiropractor sought my help because he felt overwhelmed by his patients' pain. These professionals are often independent and work alone. They are individually responsible for ensuring that their work is ethical and that they have adequate resources to deal with stress. Although an independent practitioner is free from the stress of being part of a large organisation such as the NHS, she may suffer from isolation and lack of support unless she has a secure professional network for peer support.

Patients may be ambivalent about seeking complementary treatment, and some hedge their bets by using conventional treatment as well. Practitioners may need to cooperate with other healthcare professionals when this is the case.

Care in the community

The phrase 'care in the community' was coined when reorganisation of services for the long-term mentally ill resulted in the closure of large mental hospitals. The vision was that the mentally ill could be integrated into the community and cared for in small units more closely resembling a normal living environment. In many respects this was a laudable aim. Instead of being hidden away, these patients became visible and their needs became an explicitly communal responsibility. By the same token, the staff caring for them became more visible. Perhaps the nature of the work changed in ways that were unexpected. Instead of helping to protect society from the knowledge of mental illness, carers became part of the agenda to address inequality. A new generation of workers in community care will be more likely to have this at the forefront of their conscious aims.

Care in the community also includes care of the elderly, those who are physically challenged, and children in care. In all cases professional standards and managerial responsibility must be maintained while at the same time providing a caring environment that more closely resembles a home than a hospital. In this setting it can be hard to maintain appropriate boundaries. A carer may be in danger of forgetting that she is primarily in a professional rather than a family role.

The level of managerial supervision in community settings and care homes may be low and the workload high, leading to a danger of slipping standards and tolerance of bad practice. Public and private provision exist side by side, especially in the realm of care for the elderly, and public-sector patients may be cared for in private care homes. Private care homes will have explicit business interests that may conflict with the altruistic aims of the care workers.

Care of the elderly and community care for terminally ill patients also raise the issue of endings and bereavement. The significance of fear of death and the choice of a career in caring as reparation for childhood bereavement were explored in Chapter 1. All these areas of possible conflict of interest cause extra stress. Staff will need support and understanding from managers and counsellors, bearing in mind the special demands of this sector.

Care in the community overlaps with social services, and many of the recipients of care in this sector need both medical and social care.

Social services

Development of the social work profession

Social care services evolved from charity and the Poor Laws of 1601 and 1834. Wealthy individuals and religious organisations gave to the poor and destitute. Perhaps a sense of fairness or sometimes guilt about their own good fortune lay behind this redistribution of resources. The Poor Laws were criticised because individuals only qualified for help in the district or parish where they lived, so they were discouraged from looking elsewhere for work and became stuck in dependency. If they had nowhere else to live they would be sent to the local workhouse, where as its name implies subsistence was exchanged for labour. The work and the accommodation were menial and extremely unpleasant. To be consigned to the workhouse was a terrible fate, on a par with going to prison. In a sense it was a punishment for failure or poverty. Aid was often linked to family size, and justifiably so, but there was no incentive to curtail a growing family, thus perpetuating family inadequacy. The Victorian Charity Organisation Society noted in its 1881 report[10] that the poverty of the working classes was often due to their improvident habits and thriftlessness.

Alleviation of poverty, social exclusion and deprivation increasingly became the responsibility of the State, although charities and religious establishments continued to play a part and still do so. Services for different community needs developed in parallel, resulting in a variety of titles and roles for what we now know as social workers. There was no overall training or regulation of social workers until the British Federation of Social Workers was formed in 1936. This organisation was intended to bring a sense of unity to a diverse and fragmented profession.

During the 1960s, Government commitment to addressing the problems of poverty and social exclusion led to an expansion in the ranks of social workers, but there remained a sense of lack of coordination and of being undervalued. It took the efforts of Richard Titmuss[11] and Sir Frederic (later Lord) Seebohm to create a progressive and coordinated welfare service. The implementation of the Seebohm Report[12] resulted in the formation of a new unified professional body, namely the British Association of Social Workers and also the Central Council for Education and Training in Social Work. This was a great achievement for the profession, and it gave it the status it had long desired. Sadly, the optimism and high expectations were short-lived because of the subsequent downturn in the economy. Expansion and professional status failed to bring about much change in the difficulties faced by the recipients of the welfare services and the social workers who were trying to help them.

There were several high-profile failures in the 1970s, particularly in the field of child abuse, that seriously eroded public confidence in social workers. Raised expectations made the shortcomings seem even more dramatic. One of the responses to the public enquiries that followed was to strengthen the management role of social workers. This is a further reflection of increased professional status. Trained social workers are now managers of resources, and some of the delivery of care is delegated to less experienced workers or carers. Clients are becoming empowered to have a say in their own care plans, and this also carries the understanding that they should do what they can to look after themselves. Services are provided by a range of formal and informal carers in a reversal of the earlier reforms.

We now recognise that the Welfare State cannot meet all needs. Just as with medicine, the alleviation of poverty and deprivation is an idealistic vision that is ultimately impossible to achieve by State intervention. Clients are explicitly encouraged to work out their own solutions rather than depend on others to do this for them.

Reform goes on. Legislation in 2003 entitled *Every Child Matters*[13] seeks to bring together the whole range of health, welfare, education and judicial services for children under a single umbrella. All the different agencies involved are charged with working together in a coordinated way and communicating with each other to serve the best interests of children. The underlying message has changed from child care to child protection – a shift from nurturing to control, which mirrors changes taking place elsewhere in social services.

Justice and court social work

By the end of the nineteenth century, Court Missionaries assisted magistrates in dealing with vulnerable offenders. The Missionaries were renamed Probation Officers in the Probation of Offenders Act in 1907. Their remit was to 'advise, assist and befriend' the offenders in their care. Since the Criminal Justice and Court Services Act 2000 the National Probation Service has become part of the Offender Management Service and its aims are different. The triad is now 'enforcement, rehabilitation and public protection.' This represents a significant shift in emphasis, and is more about punishment and protecting the public than about supporting the offenders. Probation officers are in the process of coming to terms with this change in ethos, which in many cases conflicts with their personal aims.

The Children and Family Court Advisory and Support Service (CAFCASS) has social workers employed by the legal system to investigate and make assessments in disputes between parents, in order to advise the courts on the best way to serve the interests of children in disrupted families. These social workers are explicitly advocates for children, but work in an atmosphere of conflict where parents are unable to agree on how to share the task of parenting. It is a skilful and difficult job to step aside from the dispute and look clearly at the needs of the children involved. Managers and counsellors supporting CAFCASS personnel will be more effective in providing support if they are aware of these conflicts and the possibility of projection and parallel process, resulting in spillover into other areas of the worker's life. These psychological processes are explored further in Chapters 2 and 5. Systems theory helps those working with families to understand how emotions may be passed around and sometimes projected on to others.

Understanding social work

There is a real challenge in working with people who are not coping with life, in a way that does not add to their problems. Social workers recognise that health, poverty and education must all be addressed in order to improve the lives of their clients, but these may be the very issues that fall by the wayside when resources are limited. The clients themselves are not always voluntary recipients of help, and may only want selected parts of the solution. A service user who is angry about her situation, whether it is disability or poverty, may vent her anger on a social worker. The social worker's desire to help may be frustrated by the failure of clients to make use of what is on offer.

Sometimes solutions may be forced upon clients – for example, if the welfare of children is at risk. Social services must by law fulfil obligations to provide child protection, so this part of the workload is outside the control of the organisation. Children and other vulnerable people may not feel empowered to ask for what they need, so it is right that they are protected by statutory provision. However, the budget is finite, so there will always be tension between the needs of the service users and the providers who have to make the best use of the available resources while at the same time meeting legal minimum standards.

There are similarities between the problems of the service users and the issues that social workers themselves find difficult to cope with. When social workers bring their concerns to support agencies, it is helpful to keep these synergies in mind. The phenomenon of parallel process was explored in Chapter 2. It can enable a worker to understand how she may become caught up in her client's problems, and to make a clearer boundary for herself. The following issues will be explored:

- confusion
- conflict
- power imbalance
- rescuing
- ambivalence
- gender
- change.

Confusion

When the social work profession was in its early stages, the idea was to work with families or individuals to identify their needs and help them to live more organised lives. Poverty, deprivation and illness often coexist. There is much debate about which of these comes first and whether the problem is the inadequacy of the social system or a client's ignorance and inability to organise herself. In reality the family system is deeply resistant to change, even if it is apparently dysfunctional. Formerly, the underlying principle of the casework relationship was that the support of a social worker would enable clients (especially families) to be rehabilitated into orderly citizens. The model was based on the assumption that families should conform to a pattern set by others, without questioning whether this was reasonable or appropriate. This interventionist approach was unpopular with clients, and they often resented the interference of social workers. Clients may not understand why they are expected to change their behaviour.

Where there is confusion there is often an impulse to put it in order, but perhaps we can now allow people to choose their own version and the degree of order that they want in their lives. Although service users may have this choice, social workers must conform to externally imposed standards of practice and statutory requirements. In other words, social workers also often experience chaos and imposed solutions. Overload and reorganisation cause additional confusion.

If there are too many things to deal with, the temptation is to do only the most important ones, or to run away, withdraw or collapse emotionally. In crisis management, priorities are determined by what causes the greatest discomfort. Managers and social workers as well as clients experience the effects of crisis management. The issues that social service employees bring to counselling and support agencies reflect feelings of overwhelming workload, confusion and disorder. Managers and staff support services may be able to help with ordering priorities or by giving permission to take time out to recover emotionally. Sometimes what managers or counsellors can offer workers who feel confused and overwhelmed by their caseload is time away from the pressure of work, to move away from crisis management, look at the reality and make a measured assessment of their conflicting priorities.

Conflict

Conflict is a thread that runs through all aspects of social care for both clients and staff. Different values, unfairness and difficult choices all cause feelings of frustration. I have already pointed out the role conflict of care versus control, with which many social workers struggle. One major source of conflict is the fact that funding for personal social services comes largely from local government rather than from central government. Because of this, the service users are geographically closer to the decision makers and sometimes become very vocal about their priorities.

Social services compete for funding with other services. Local councils have the difficult job of allocating limited resources to a range of equally deserving causes. When the choice is between funding care homes for the elderly or services for physically or mentally disabled people, one group or the other is likely to be disappointed. It may be very difficult for the professionals to contain their own frustration, and the clients are even more likely to let their anger spill over. This is just one example of the opposing forces that have to be kept in balance in order to carry on with the job. Anger management skills may be needed as part of the support provided for both clients and social workers.

Power imbalance

Social workers may struggle with the conflict between wanting to offer help and empowering clients to make their own choice about what help they need. The work of conducting assessments and allocating limited resources may feel uncomfortably like denial of help. If help is offered too readily, an individual cannot develop the skill of looking after her own needs. This is one of the essential steps in becoming a competent adult. Just as a parent's job is to nurture and support children to do this in the safety of the family, a social worker may feel that she is in a parental role in relation to her clients when trying to encourage independence. Yet she is not their parent, and she must take care not to abuse the power of her role. Social workers bear a heavy responsibility when using the power to give or withhold help.

Clients find it harder to accept advice when there is a power imbalance. There is a natural antipathy to accepting help when it is offered in a 'we know best' spirit. This is almost guaranteed to bring out the 'rebellious child' response – to do the opposite of what is desired! Or it may confirm the recipient's sense of inadequacy and failure, perpetuating feelings of degradation and disillusionment rather than helping to eradicate them. Social workers often feel frustrated and inadequate just as their clients do. Social workers must also learn how to get their own needs met, and may need help with this. Managers and counsellors will not be able to remove the problems, but may be able to help to put them in perspective.

Rescuing

Many social work clients seem to be victims. Life has given them a raw deal. The Welfare State was set up to redress the balance and provide help for people who need it – in other words, to rescue them. Social workers are professional rescuers.

Compulsive carers (*see* Chapter 1) are rescuers. The roles of victim and rescuer belong to a dynamic that also includes the role of persecutor. This is known as the 'drama triangle' (*see* Figure 3.1), as described by Karpman.[14]

Those who participate in the drama exchange roles from time to time, but the drama perpetuates a situation of power imbalance that seems to have no solution. A social worker who tries to rescue a client may prevent that client from learning to fend for herself. In this way she disempowers her client and becomes a persecutor rather than a rescuer, and the client remains stuck in victim mode. If the client does not make good use of the proffered help, or relapses into chaotic behaviour, the social worker may begin to feel like a victim who is being persecuted by a difficult client, and she may hope to be rescued by her manager. All of those involved may perceive that they are victims of the inadequacy of the welfare system. The effect of these roles is to inhibit change. The value of a drama is that the exchange of roles gives the appearance of doing something, but the underlying problems persist. It constitutes a defence against facing difficult emotions. When a victim is willing to give up her stereotyped role and find another way to manage her life, the situation may improve. At least she will be making her own decisions and taking more responsibility. If a social worker can offer help towards constructive solutions without taking control, she may avoid the disempowering effect of rescuing.

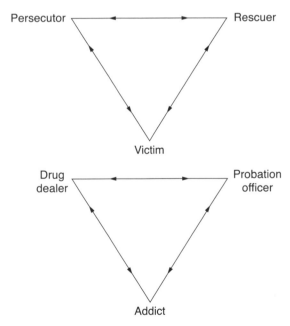

Figure 3.1 The drama triangle. *Source*: Karpman S (1968) Fairy tales and script drama analysis. *Trans Anal Bull.* **9**: 39–43. (To view article *see* www.KarpmanDramaTriangle.com.)

Drug addicts are often seen as victims. Their actions seem to be controlled by the need to get the next fix. They may be persecuted by drug suppliers or by the police who arrest them when they commit offences to feed their habit. People from whom they steal also feel persecuted. Courts now often combine punishment with a drug rehabilitation requirement. Probation officers who administer the rehabilitation programme recognise that they can easily be cast in the role of a rescuer or a persecutor, but the programme is only effective if the addict is willing to take responsibility for their own actions and make the decision to kick their habit.

The drama triangle is a device that allows people to blame others for their problems, and this prevents progress. When the protagonists decide to stop playing roles and choose a more effective way forward, progress is possible. It only takes one of the role players to break the cycle. If there is no persecutor, there is no victim and no need for a rescuer. If there is no rescuer, the victim must learn to be self-sufficient. However, it is not necessarily easy for victims to avoid persecution. Drug addicts have been known to ask for a prison sentence to put them out of reach of dealers.

Counsellors, managers and other support workers can easily join in the drama unless they are self-aware and properly supervised. Supervision can enable a counsellor or social worker to stop their own role in the drama triangle and thus benefit the person they are trying to help. Supervision is explored further in Chapter 5.

Ambivalence

The piecemeal development of different strands of social services resulted in a fragmented service with little sense of professional solidarity. The work of social services takes place in a variety of locations serving several different sections of the community, including children and families, mental health patients, the court service and care of the elderly. Often these groups are on the margins of society. Many are in the process of transition – from hospital to care in the community, from independence to needing support, or from prison to the outside world. Their confusion and insecurity are mirrored by social workers who often feel that they too are at the periphery of society, and provide a link from the unacceptable to the acceptable face of society.

Social workers deal with the aspects of life that many of us find uncomfortable. Part of their function may be to protect the rest of the community from facing unpleasant reality. This may make life easier for those who are already comfortable, but it is debatable whether it makes much difference to the lives of service users. Some argue that social workers subconsciously expect, and are expected by others, to take on the task of absolving society's collective guilt about inequality.

A psychological split may occur between the acceptable and the unacceptable. This phenomenon explains why an individual may deny unwanted character traits, and sometimes attribute or project them on to other individuals in an attempt to resolve confusion. It sometimes happens in organisations and in the community. A social worker, whose job title indicates that she is willing to shoulder society's problems, may become the container for the negativity felt by society about poverty and deprivation. She may become a scapegoat and be blamed whenever anything goes wrong. Child protection officers are a vivid example of how this can happen.

In the inquiry into the Cleveland child abuse cases,[15] social workers and doctors were accused of intervening too readily in cases of suspected child abuse when there was inadequate evidence. On the other hand, if child abuse is ignored because the evidence is not taken sufficiently seriously, there may be tragic consequences for the child, as in the Victoria Climbie case.[16] Families resent interference. If social workers hold back from investigating suspected child abuse and children are hurt, they are castigated. However, if they accuse innocent parents of abuse, they are perceived to be inept and intrusive. If they quietly get on with the job, no one even notices them.

Social workers are often in a highly ambivalent position, as they are meant to offer support to families while at the same time they have a role in reporting abuse or neglect of children. Parents may sometimes regard them with fear and suspicion. The role conflict of 'friend or spy' coupled with the stress of the consequences of making a wrong decision creates a difficult burden for the child protection officer to carry. Social work managers also find role conflict familiar. As well as the ambivalence of their role for clients, managers are also in an ambivalent relationship with their team members. A team manager must ensure that members of staff are performing their statutory duties properly while at the same time offering support and understanding when the workload seems overwhelming and difficult decisions have to be made. She has to balance care and control for the staff in her team.

Gender

In the context of family support it is worth considering the gender aspects of social work. The role of the social worker is in many respects similar to the role of women and especially mothers in a traditional family. Mothers do the caring and many of the less appealing tasks for the rest of the family, get the blame if things go wrong, and receive very little thanks! Now this is an old-fashioned view of motherhood and family life, and the situation is gradually changing for social workers and for families, but some cages are being rattled in the process. Traditional role models are part of the stable family system that is resistant to change. It can function well, but it may not suit the modern concept of sexual equality. The tasks of family life are now more equitably shared by men and women in many homes.

More men are joining the caring professions. When social work was undergoing reform and regulation to become a more professional service, one of the results was an increase in the number of men entering the profession. However, men are concentrated in the managerial ranks whereas women are still more likely to be the deliverers of care. Sexual equality has not been fully achieved, but the situation is gradually changing for the better.

Change

Organisational change was explored in Chapter 2. Social workers have to face organisational change and at the same time help their clients to deal with their changing circumstances.

Radical changes in management philosophy are a feature of the social work profession, as they are for the NHS. Crisis, conflict and change are recurring themes in social work and have been so from the very beginning. These are the same issues that the clients and users of social services are struggling with as well. Social workers may empathise with their clients when change is imposed from above and people who are far removed from the detail seem to know what should be done to improve the service. Like other professional carers, social workers resist change and prefer to do things their own way.

Often workers engage with the process of modernisation and recognise that it is unrealistic to expect to stand still, but eventually imposed and repeated change wears them down. Then a seemingly trivial change, such as a new boss, a move of office or a colleague going off sick, may be the catalyst for loss of control and inability to cope. New opportunities bring frustration and anxiety as well as benefits. Sometimes it is easier to carry on with imperfect but familiar patterns of behaviour than to learn new methods. As social workers support families or individuals coping with change, they need empathy, encouragement and positive reframing from managers and support services when organisational change occurs.

Charities

It is now explicit that management of resources for social care includes the charity sector. There is a long history of charitable support for vulnerable members of society, pre-dating any government provision. It is still the case that members of the public wish to help by giving time and money to help those who need it. Many of the issues about management, training and hierarchy are the same for charities as for other care providers. It is no longer acceptable to rely on good intentions. The rules of the Charity Commission ensure the probity of registered charities, and charity workers must have professional standards and proper procedures to protect both clients and workers.

Often volunteers do virtually identical work to those in the paid sector – for example, in counselling, children's services or hospice care. There is no guaranteed funding for charities, and part of the job is often to raise funds as well as to provide services. Voluntary workers may not be able to pay for their own training – indeed they may have chosen to do charity work for this reason. If individuals are expected to work to professional standards, many will expect to be paid at a professional rate for the job. Some charities have both voluntary and paid staff. Managers often have the difficult task of juggling the conflicting demands of professional standards and voluntary workers. In addition, volunteers are dedicated but sometimes fickle. One of the attractions of charity work is its flexibility. The worker has much more freedom to work or not to work as it suits her. The manager has to organise all of this into a coherent and credible service.

Supporting charity workers is just as vital as supporting paid workers. It is as well to remember that the subconscious contract may take a number of different forms here. The employer wants a high standard of care and dedicated commitment. The worker may want various things, including training, flexibility, appeasement of the pain of her own bereavement, companionship, or the feeling of 'making a difference.' Support services may have to address these issues as well as the expected strains of the work. In recognition of the fact that the work is unpaid, support services for staff in the voluntary sector are sometimes better than those for workers in paid employment.

Professional discipline

Employees in health and social care are subject to professional standards, personal benefits, disciplinary procedures and the possible effects of discrimination. These issues affect them as individuals, but are put into practice and regulated by the employing organisations and professional bodies.

Professional standards

Established professions such as medicine, nursing and social work have evolved over many decades. People who performed the same kind of work started to be known by certain labels. Descriptive labels changed as the nature of the job changed, or as fashions changed. Almoners, or dispensers of alms, became social workers. Distributing alms is not what they do any more. Barbers became surgeons. Now surgeons are subdivided into specialties according to which parts of the body they operate on. Groups of professionals exchanged or shared information and defined their areas of expertise. This expertise became a precious commodity that had to be protected, so entry to the group became a privilege restricted to those who fulfilled certain criteria. Once entry is restricted, a select group is needed to set entry conditions and determine who can join. Members must continue to meet the prescribed standards in order to maintain the security and the reputation of the group. Professional standards are also important for protecting the users of the services.

Some professions are self-regulating, setting their own standards, with the professional association acting as the regulatory body. Arguably only those within the profession are qualified to judge whether or not professional standards are being upheld. The General Medical Council (GMC) is such a body. However, the conflict of interest between upholding standards and protecting its members has resulted in its reputation being seriously undermined. In some cases the interests of members have been protected at the expense of the safety of the users. The constitution of the GMC has been changed so that it now has a majority of non-medical members. The public rightly expects that it should receive treatment or care that meets the accepted standard. When it does not it will complain and want redress.

Social workers are regulated and registered by the General Social Care Council in the UK, as required by the Care Standards Act 2000. Counselling, psychotherapy and other therapies are in the process of coming under statutory regulation. In recognition of the importance of this for the protection of the public, most of the individual health and social care professions have already established their own regulatory bodies – for example, the British Association for Counselling and Psychotherapy (BACP). Members of professions allied to medicine may be registered with the Health Professions Council. This body sets standards of professional training, performance and conduct for a range of health professions.

There are many ways for a counsellor to qualify. In the past it was possible to become a counsellor with little formal training. Many counsellors have had a previous career, often in another of the human professions, such as nursing or teaching. They may have developed counselling skills in other walks of life and then decide to formally train to be a counsellor, as I did. Regulation of professional standards now requires formal training and maintenance of expertise by ongoing professional development. A degree or diploma course in counselling or psychology may be followed by further academic study for an MSc. BACP accredits counsellor training courses that meet its standards, and accredits counsellors who have reached the required standard. The training and professional ethics of counsellors are regulated for the protection of both practitioners and clients. Registration of counsellors is administered by the United Kingdom Register of Counsellors.

Individuals have a personal responsibility to ensure that they are fit to practise, but upholding professional standards is also part of the remit of staff support services. If workers become too stressed they may lose their competence and their sense of perspective. Sometimes it is necessary for occupational health professionals or counsellors to insist that workers take time out, so that their safety or that of the patients or clients is not compromised. BACP requires registered counsellors to have regular supervision, and the British Medical Association recommends doctors to take steps to reduce their stress levels as part of their continuing professional development.

Professional standards are important, but the setting of high standards is a double-edged sword. Of course recipients of care should expect to be treated with expertise and respect, but when things go wrong they look for someone to blame. We live in what is called a 'blame culture', where it no longer seems acceptable for accidents to occur. Psychologically the pain of a disaster is lessened if someone can be held accountable. Fear of litigation may certainly keep professionals on their toes with regard to following correct procedures and accurately documenting what they do. However, it also leads to defensive activity, such as tests that are of questionable value to the patient, and it adds another burden of stress to health and social care professionals.

Complaints and professional negligence claims

Complaints and negligence claims have a profound and damaging effect on professionals, even when claims are not upheld. Those who label themselves experts in counselling, social work or medicine gain prestige and hopefully respect from their professional status, but also set themselves up for a fall when blame is to be apportioned.

Patients who feel that they have been wrongly treated or that they have been damaged by their treatment have the right to complain to the organisation responsible for their treatment, or to the professional body of the individual about whom they are complaining. A member of staff may be aggrieved by the behaviour of a colleague, and also has the right to complain. Various procedures will be brought into effect, depending on the type and seriousness of the complaint. In addition to the complainant and the accused, the management or organisation may also come under scrutiny. Blame may be passed up the line to the people who gave the instructions or set the policies.

Sometimes it appears that expectation of redress drives a compensation culture that encourages personal injury litigation. Many victims of negligence claim that they only want an apology, or to prevent anything similar happening again, but then get caught up in an adversarial process with a momentum that can get out of control. Prolonged investigations may generate further distress and anger.

If the problem can be put in perspective, so that small issues are dealt with informally or by mediation, before jumping into an official complaints procedure, it is often possible to defuse a situation before it escalates. This is less damaging for the people involved and may result in a quicker resolution. However, it is important not to belittle complaints, and proper procedures must be in place, and must be used if informal measures do not resolve the problem. Human resources departments and counselling services sometimes work together to provide mediation and resolution of grievances.

The effects of investigations into professional misconduct are devastating for all the individuals concerned. All of those affected become victims of the system. Often it will not be clear who is at fault. How can we blame a social worker for losing track of a child when she cannot gain access to the child's home to make checks, or she is overloaded with casework and cannot possibly spend the necessary time with every child on her case list? Is her manager to blame? Is the local government authority to blame for not allocating sufficient resources, or the taxpayer for being unwilling to pay more tax?

Sometimes cases take years to reach a conclusion. The injured party remains in a state of suspended animation, often unable to grieve or move on until the case has been resolved. An accused professional is usually immediately suspended pending investigation. She cannot work and may be forbidden to communicate with colleagues. The effect of even a minor complaint on an individual's confidence can be severe.[17] Suspension is particularly hard for a professional who relies on her work as a coping strategy, or as a source of self-esteem. She may face long empty days in which to brood over her anxieties while the investigations proceed. Offloading by talking to friends or colleagues is another recognised way of releasing stress, but she may not be allowed to do this. People who appear to be strong and competent professionals can suddenly find themselves undermined and at a loss to know how to cope. Asking for help may be an unfamiliar and very difficult thing to do. The caregiver has to face her own unexpected vulnerability. Counsellors have a vital role in supporting those involved in disciplinary procedures, but must be aware of possible conflicts of interest and the legal limits of confidentiality. BACP gives guidance on professional conduct for counsellors, and also on legal disclosure of information obtained during counselling.

Bullying

Bullying is often a response to stress. Bullies wish to appear strong and capable but may feel insecure. Instead of resolving feelings of inadequacy, some people cope by trying to exert power over those whom they perceive to be weaker. This may be by physical intimidation, gang culture (there is safety in numbers), or by belittling and undermining them verbally. It is especially prevalent in hierarchical environments such as hospitals and schools. In the *Working Well Survey* by the Royal College of Nursing[18] it was found that 17% of respondents had been bullied by another member of staff during the year before the survey.

The hierarchy in hospitals continues to allow consultants a degree of autonomy that makes it difficult to challenge inappropriate behaviour. However, bullying is unacceptable and should be challenged until the culture changes. Bullying of junior doctors by consultants is sometimes seen as a rite of passage and a necessary 'toughening up' process, but an atmosphere of intimidation is not conducive to learning and can result in disillusionment and loss of confidence. After working for one such consultant, a junior doctor said to me 'Now I am going to take six months' unpaid leave to recover my strength.' Junior doctors are particularly unwilling to complain because they fear jeopardising the reference that will further their career. Mostly it is easier to keep their head down, knowing that they will soon move on to another job. Thus the problem continues and becomes part of the culture. Sometimes the bullied go on to bully others when the role model has been set. It is important for managers to ensure that appropriate anti-bullying policies are in place. Support services may be called upon to offer help to both parties by mediation, counselling and appropriate assertiveness training.

The politics of bullying

Occasionally bullying comes from higher in the system. The setting of targets for political reasons may have this effect. Targets are an effective way of focusing on priorities and ensuring that revenue is spent efficiently. If the targets are un-realistic or impossible to achieve, staff may feel pressurised to cut corners or falsify results in order to satisfy the target setters. There are many examples of the adverse effects of unrealistic goals. Workers who are unable to do the job properly due to inadequate resources lose job satisfaction and become disillusioned. Cleaning contracts that are under-resourced result in dirty hospitals and high rates of infection. It is often those at the bottom of the hierarchy who suffer when they have no one to whom to delegate.

Waiting, and waiting

A clerk in the surgical waiting-list office was devastated when he found that some patients had been waiting too long for operations, and his department was severely criticised for failing to meet Government targets. There was no clear system of priorities, and some patients waited longer than others for no good reason. He had been involved in sending letters to or telephoning some of these patients, and felt personally responsible for their pain. He had been following instructions from his manager, who in turn was taking orders from the surgeons.

It can be difficult to know who is responsible in situations like this. The most vulnerable person in the chain may take on the stress for the whole system. With the support of an Employee Assistance Programme (EAP) counsellor this employee was able to put his role into perspective and to feel more able to speak out in future if he felt that what he was being asked to do was unfair.

Discrimination

Consistent with the spectrum of health and illness in the population, it is statistically likely that some professional carers will have health issues. Can staff with chronic mental or physical illness or disability work effectively? Arguably a care professional who has health needs is more likely to understand the needs of others. Health and social care employers must, like all employers, adhere to the legal requirements of the Disability Discrimination Act and the Equal Opportunities Act. This means that reasonable provision must be made to enable disabled staff to remain at work.

At times support agencies may be asked to help staff who are experiencing discrimination. Discrimination can be subtle and internalised as part of the culture – for example, by use of language or context. Workers may present for help with stress that they do not immediately associate with discrimination. It is only when the problem is explored in more depth that it becomes apparent what is happening.

Cold feet

Ginny, a social worker for an asylum-seekers project, developed health problems. Arthritis and poor circulation affected her ability to work. She took to wearing thick boots and extra layers of clothing to alleviate her discomfort in a cold office. When she had several episodes of sick leave she was referred for counselling. She felt angry because she was unable to do for herself what she aimed to do for her clients – to enable them to access services to live as normal a life as possible. She worked in an office in an outpost where the heating was inadequate and there were no support staff nearby.

She realised that she had allowed herself to become marginalised just as her clients were. The solutions that her manager offered were a portable heater and a time switch, not a move to a better office. The worker became the problem due to her medical complaints. Only the symptoms were addressed, not the underlying discrimination.

Racial diversity in health and social care

When the solution to the post-war labour shortage was addressed by encouraging emigration from Commonwealth countries, healthcare was one of the main sectors to benefit. Nurses and doctors from Caribbean countries and the Indian subcontinent helped to make up the shortfall in the UK. There is now a new staff crisis in healthcare, due partly to disillusionment causing staff to leave, but also due to the fact that there is a shortage of trained staff in a whole variety of occupations. Care workers have more choice, and leave to take a different job if they are dissatisfied where they are. Technical advances in healthcare and changes such as the European working-time directive mean that more staff are needed than before. Recruits can easily move about Europe to find work, and also many professionals migrate from Malaysia, Eastern Europe and Africa to fill vacancies in the NHS. Refugees often have valuable skills and are eager to work, but need help to complete the professional registration requirements.

Hospitals provide induction courses, accommodation and training to help foreign workers to settle in and integrate with their new surroundings. However, it is still common for immigrants to feel isolated, homesick or misunderstood, and they seek help from staff support services for these issues. Often they cope well until some unforeseen event such as illness strikes them. As their family and friends are far away they do not have the usual personal support systems available to them, and they may need additional help and understanding from staff support services.

Staff benefits

Working for a large public-sector employer has advantages for the worker. Every town and city and even small communities have health and social care workers. There are job opportunities at every level, including children's services, personal care, district nurses, health visitors, health centre staff, and so on. There is usually work available for people who want to work locally and with flexible hours. 'Return to nursing' courses help nurses who have taken a career break to get back to their professional work. Banks of secretarial and nursing staff enable matching of those available to work flexibly with changes in service needs. Lack of qualifications is often no barrier, as training is provided and there will also be opportunities to gain qualifications on the job. Promotion prospects are good for those who want to advance themselves.

Doctors benefit from high rates of pay, opportunities for professional development, and public esteem. Flexible working is available at all career levels.

Working in health and social care may convey a sense of safety. Workers may feel they should be cared for as well as the clients or patients. Just as there is a subconscious expectation of care between the carer and the patient 'I will care for you and make you better', there is sometimes a subconscious expectation of care between the organisation and the staff. This applies to all staff, not just those working in direct contact with clients. Secretaries, cleaners, maintenance staff and others all seem to feel safer when they work in a caring environment. However, sometimes these expectations of care are unrealistic and the perks may be no better than in any other job. Traditionally healthcare offered job security, but organisational changes mean that this is no longer guaranteed. As a result there are feelings of insecurity and disillusionment among some groups.

Provision of a staff support service is an important acknowledgement that an organisation does value and care for its employees. Sensitive management and peer support will help, but it is also necessary to provide confidential help that is not directly linked to the worker's colleagues. This benefit can be provided in different ways, and more information about the range of staff support services can be found in Chapter 5.

Summary

The general principles of organisational practice have been applied to the different bodies that deliver health and social care, and the ways in which these may affect individuals who work in these sectors have been examined.

The NHS and social services are large public organisations responsible for delivering most of the health and social care in the UK. Their cultural characteristics have evolved over the years. Early in their history, development was unstructured and inconsistent, but during the twentieth and early twenty-first centuries politically driven change has imposed control and attempted to make the provision of care fairer and more consistent. Health and social care are now consumer led and subject to market forces.

In healthcare there is an explicit awareness of the cost of services, and Government expects efficient and cost-effective use of resources. This sometimes causes staff to feel that they must concentrate on productivity at the expense of compassionate care. Hospitals are adopting more flexible working practices to cope with these new demands. Primary care services are also under pressure from their users' expectations of a rapid response to a wide range of health problems. Primary care is at the interface between specialist healthcare, care in the community and social services. The difficulty of being in this buffer zone, and often acting as advocates or gatekeepers for other services, creates additional tensions for workers and managers.

Care professionals in the private sector and complementary medicine face similar stresses to other care workers, in that compulsive caring, overwhelming demands, ambivalence and conflicting values are likely to occur from time to time. In these sectors professional isolation is a danger, and professional regulation is less well developed.

Care in the community enables those who are not able to live independently to enjoy a lifestyle that more closely resembles a home, instead of living in an institution. The care workers who help clients to live in this way are neither relatives nor nurses, and must remain aware of the need to maintain appropriate boundaries. Sometimes they are faced with the progressive decline or death of a client. This work is often challenging, and carers will need support from managers and counsellors to overcome the difficulties.

Social care is aimed at alleviating poverty and deprivation, especially for vulnerable people. This is a huge task that often feels overwhelming for workers. They are sometimes blamed individually when tragedies result from systemic failures. Many social workers are uncomfortable with the fact that the underlying ethos of their work has changed from care to an uneasy balance of care and control. Unconscious psychological processes are often operating, and social workers can easily be drawn into the dynamics of persecutor, victim and rescuer, the so-called 'drama triangle.'

Lack of resources and the increasing expectations of clients are also issues for the voluntary sector of health and social care. Here managers integrate paid and unpaid workers and take account of the different motivation of volunteers. They must also use their resources effectively and adhere to the requirements of regulatory bodies such as the Charity Commission.

Professional regulatory bodies have evolved from organisations designed to protect the interests of their members, to defining and upholding standards of practice and protecting the public from the effects of malpractice. The interests of members may sometimes conflict with the interests of the public, so we now have to consider whether such bodies can adequately perform all of these functions. Workers are put under enormous stress when service users complain, or if they are accused of malpractice. Managers and staff support services are often called upon to help employees to cope with the resulting investigations. These can be protracted, adding further to the burden of stress.

Individuals have a personal responsibility to ensure that they are fit to practise. Managers and counsellors may have to remind employees of this responsibility if they believe that their fitness for safe and ethical practice may be compromised.

Ethical practice for employers includes a duty to ensure that bullying and other forms of unfair discrimination do not occur in the working environment. The necessary policies should be in place, and if any incidents do occur, appropriate measures should be taken, including disciplinary action, counselling and training.

There are many benefits to working in the caring professions. A huge number and variety of jobs are available in this sector, from highly skilled professionals to support staff in grades that require few formal qualifications. There are opportunities to gain new skills, and flexible working practices are common. Job satisfaction is generally high, despite the many difficulties encountered. In recognition of the fact that the work is stressful, most employers provide a staff support service as a benefit of employment. Chapter 4 looks at the range of issues for which staff seek help, and Chapter 5 describes the different ways in which support may be provided.

References

1 Beveridge W (1942) *The Beveridge Report. Social Insurance and Allied Services.* HMSO, London.
2 Illich I (1975) *Medical Nemesis.* Calder and Boyars, London.
3 Griffiths R (1983) *NHS Management Report.* Department of Health and Social Security, London.
4 Secretary of State for Health (1989) *Working for Patients.* HMSO, London.
5 Department of Health (1992) *The Health of the Nation.* Department of Health, London.
6 Department of Health (1995) *The Patients' Charter Revised and Expanded.* Department of Health, London.
7 NHS Institute for Innovation and Improvement; www.institute.nhs.uk
8 Caplan RP (1994) Stress, anxiety and depression in hospital consultants, general practitioners and senior health service managers. *BMJ.* **309:** 1261–3.
9 Brewin CR and Firth-Cozens J (1997) Dependency and self-criticism as predictors of depression in young doctors. *J Occ Health Psychol.* **2**(3): 242-6.
10 Victorian Charity Organisation Society (1881) *Review. Volume 10.* Victorian Charity Organisation Society, London.
11 Titmuss RM (1965) Goals of today's Welfare State. In: P Anderson and R Blackburn (eds) *Towards Socialism.* Fontana, London.
12 Seebohm F (1968) *Seebohm Report of the Committee on Local Authority and Allied Personal Social Services.* HMSO, London.
13 Department of Health (2003) *Every Child Matters.* The Stationery Office, London.
14 Karpman S (1968) Fairy tales and script drama analysis. *Transact Anal Bull.* **9:** 39–43.
15 Butler-Sloss E (1987) *Report of the Inquiry into Child Abuse in Cleveland.* HMSO, London.
16 Laming H (2003) *The Victoria Climbie Inquiry.* Department of Health, London.
17 Anon (1998) Whistleblowing or professional assassination. Personal View *BMJ.* **316:** 1756.
18 Royal College of Nursing (2002) *Working Well Survey.* Royal College of Nursing, London.

Chapter 4

Work-related stress

Introduction

There is plenty of scope for stress and misunderstanding in health and social care. Professional carers have complex aspirations and needs, and they work in organisations that have a range of organisational cultures and systems. Change and conflicting values are often prevalent. Unspoken and unknown expectations on both sides may remain unfulfilled, and in some cases it is impossible to fulfil them. This chapter explores the effects of these stresses and the ways in which they impact on professional carers.

I shall explore how people normally deal with stress by means of a range of social and psychological coping strategies. If these strategies fail, symptoms of stress occur. I shall also explain the symptoms and signs of stress and the physiology of the adrenalin cycle. Sometimes professional carers ask for help when they experience symptoms of stress, but if nothing is done to improve the situation, things may get worse until it is impossible to ignore the problems, and breakdown or burnout may result. If an employee is unable to recognise that she is having difficulty, she may be advised to get help by occupational health advisers or her GP. Colleagues or relatives may also point her in the direction of help. Stress, anxiety, burnout, the use of psychological defence mechanisms and substance abuse will also be examined in this chapter.

Both personal and organisational factors may cause stress, and often problems need to be addressed from both a personal and an organisational perspective. I shall show how professional carers cannot be treated in isolation from their working environment. Case histories illustrate how stress may arise from issues that are inherent in the work of health and social care.

In my own practice, I find that there is often more than one psychological process going on, so it is important to look beyond the presenting symptoms to see what else may be contributing to the problem. Every call for help from a distressed staff member is unique. However, there are some common themes that crop up repeatedly in various disguises. These case histories also show how interventions from managers and counsellors may make a difference. Chapter 5 goes on to explain in more detail how staff support services benefit professional carers.

Stress

Stress is a fashionable complaint, and almost a badge of success in a frenzied world: 'My stress is worse than yours!' It is accepted as normal to be stressed, but this may take people dangerously close to the margin, where another small crisis will tip them off balance. When events inside or outside the body exceed the physiological resources available to respond to them, the result is a sensation of stress.

Stress is normal

The stresses that we can expect to encounter in daily life come from a variety of sources, and are relevant to everyone, including health and social care workers. They include the following:

- environmental stress (e.g. excessive noise, heat, cold, passive smoking)
- physical tiredness
- ill health
- financial worries
- family relationships
- conflict of spiritual or moral values.

Whereas the physiological response to stress is the release of adrenalin, the conscious response is to choose a coping strategy. This may be straightforward, such as removing the source of irritation, taking a break, or getting medical help for illness. More complicated problems may need to be discussed with family or colleagues in order to negotiate a solution. These coping strategies are second nature for many people, who thereby manage to keep their stress level under control. Factors such as difficulty in saying 'no' or poor time management can sometimes be helped by assertiveness training or other behavioural strategies. If the selected response is effective, the signs of arousal due to adrenalin diminish, but if the response is ineffective, arousal continues and the feeling of stress increases.

Physiology of stress

The symptoms of stress are produced by the impact of the hormone adrenalin on various organs in the body. The adrenal glands produce adrenalin constantly but in variable quantities, which are determined by internal and external stimuli to the central nervous system and subsequently the pituitary gland. The pituitary gland secretes hormones that act upon the adrenal glands, forming a continuous feedback loop. If the supply of adrenalin is too low or does not increase in response to stimuli, the body is unable to cope with emergencies or the ups and downs of daily life. This system enables the body to mobilise resources for the response of 'fight, flight or freeze.' Adrenalin is vital for the body, and people who suffer from diseases of the adrenal or pituitary glands depend on regular medication to keep them alive.

Adrenalin causes an increase in heart rate and a rise in blood pressure. The blood supply to skeletal muscle increases, but the supply to the digestive system is reduced. These changes prepare the body for action, and are perceived as a racing pulse, anxiety, and sometimes chest discomfort. Changes in the digestive system may give a sensation of nausea or abdominal cramp, which is sometimes described as gut-wrenching. Alterations in blood flow result in heavy breathing and sweating. If the fight or flight response is frustrated, a state of suspense occurs until the physiological changes subside.

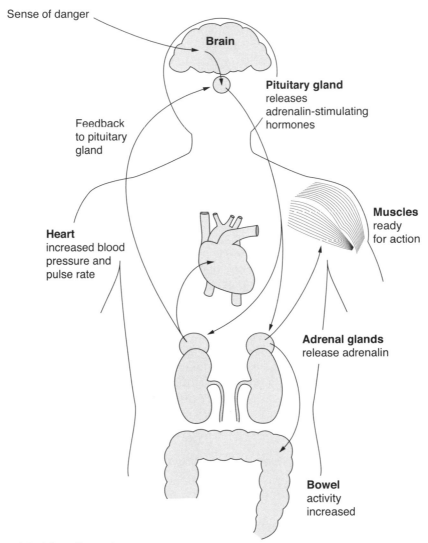

Figure 4.1 Adrenalin pathways.

Consequences of stress

Some degree of stress is essential to life. It is what keeps us going, drives ambition and motivates success. People who enter the health and social care professions do have a sense of the difficulty of the work that lies ahead. They are prepared for challenges in what they hope will be a worthwhile job. They expect the following:

- a long period of training
- physical and emotional hard work
- the need to deal with life-and-death or other difficult problems
- the need to maintain professional competence.

Too much stress has a damaging effect. If the body is in a continual state of alert, the result is anxiety, high blood pressure, heart disease and muscular weakness.

Prolonged stress depletes the body's ability to fight infection. When stress is unrelenting, instead of being ready for action the responses become paralysed and the individual is unable to cope with life. This is the point at which some people seek help or are referred for help. They may have reached a point where they are unable to make decisions for themselves, resulting in emotional and physical breakdown. Others remain aware of their own bodily reactions and, recognising that they are under increasing stress, seek help before they reach this stage. Previous experience may have taught them that it is better to stop the downward spiral before it gets out of control.

Burnout

Burnout, which has been described by Pines and Aronsen,[1] is a state of mental or physical exhaustion caused by excessive and prolonged stress. It is the result of a progression from expected and manageable pressure to unremitting and unresolved problems until the body is no longer able to respond effectively to the demands of daily life. The symptoms of burnout include being unable to face going to work, inability to make decisions, unpredictable outbursts of emotion such as crying or anger, loss of empathy, and cynicism. These are very similar to the symptoms of depression. As well as the damage to personal confidence, a worker suffering from burnout cannot work effectively and may make mistakes.

An overstressed worker may consult her doctor about depression and a variety of other medical symptoms of a psychosomatic nature. It is sometimes easier to report medical problems than emotional distress. An aware GP will check out the symptoms for physical disease and will also offer appropriate psychological treatment. Occupational health physicians may be alerted if employees have recurrent or prolonged sickness absence. These events may trigger referral to a counsellor.

Health and social care workers are especially vulnerable to burnout because of the personality traits that underlie their decision to enter the caring professions in the first place. The links between personality and career choice were considered in Chapter 1.

Personal risk factors for burnout

These include the following:

- perfectionism
- a need to be in control
- an exaggerated sense of responsibility
- difficulty in asking for help
- feelings of guilt
- suppression of emotions
- difficulty taking time out for leisure, holidays, etc.
- keeping up with advances in knowledge.

Many of these characteristics are important and necessary for the work of professional carers. Attention to detail, getting things right and being well organised are vital when dealing with life-threatening situations, or making decisions that are going to have a critical impact on a person's life. Health and social care workers often work in environments where they are pressurised to make decisions, and may not have the opportunity to consult or share the process with colleagues, so they learn to be independent and to shut out anxiety. Independent working also means that they carry more responsibility when things go wrong. It is difficult to maintain a boundary between necessary and excessive perfectionism. When the workload is high it is always tempting to stay at work longer and to avoid taking time off. Professionals must also continually update their knowledge and skills, and this is an extra demand on their time. Advances in knowledge mean that there is a need for continuing professional development, but this can also be taken to imply that the worker is never good enough.

Stan's story illustrates several features from the above list.

Stan's accident

Stan has 25 years' experience as a paramedic. He was referred to the staff counselling service by his manager after he had mistakenly used an incorrect piece of equipment during resuscitation of a patient. This was the first time he could recall making a mistake. In the event the patient survived and came to no harm as a result of his error, but he was unable to forgive himself. He was emotionally and physically shattered, and unable to work for two days because of abdominal pain and vomiting. Only his immediate colleagues were aware of what had happened. He had not told his wife about the event. 'I don't do emotion', he said.

He told the counsellor that he fully expected to be sacked, or at least to be severely disciplined. Instead his colleagues and his manager were understanding and felt that he was sufficiently experienced to learn from his mistake, and could still be trusted to do his job. The people around him behaved as if nothing had happened.

He said he would have preferred to be punished, as this would enable him to wipe the slate clean and move on.

Stan was a perfectionist, doing a highly stressful job day in, day out. When he made a mistake he had an exaggerated sense of guilt. His immediate symptoms of breakdown were accompanied by bodily symptoms of a stomach upset. In a way his distress was a form of self-punishment. Possibly also being 'sent' for counselling felt like punishment, as he would be expected to do something he did not find easy, namely to talk about his feelings. He felt that he must be in control of his emotions, and found it difficult to share his feelings even with those closest to him. His colleagues reinforced and colluded with this attitude, although his manager recognised that it might be easier for him to speak to a counsellor who was not part of his usual environment.

Counselling served the function of allowing Stan to get things off his chest by talking about the event. He spoke about his guilt and his need to feel that he had taken some punishment. He was able to recognise himself as only human and fallible. Nevertheless he remarked that he would check his equipment even more carefully in future.

Psychological defences

Psychological defences of denial, splitting and projection are vital tools for coping with overwhelming emotions. We could not manage without their protection as a short-term strategy. Alcohol and other substance abuse is frequently used as a defence against stress. When life brings continued and relentless stress, as happens for many care workers, it is necessary to have ways of offloading and more robust methods of self-protection.

Denial

Fineman[2] found that for social workers the dominant method of coping with stress was internalisation, or bottling up of emotions. Anger is one of the many possible emotional responses to stress. The problem is that anger is a forbidden emotion for many people, especially in the supposedly gentle caring professions. When anger is felt and there is no way to express it, the defence of denial may come into play. Sometimes projection comes in useful, if a situation occurs that allows the angry person to accuse someone else of being angry instead. This can be easy to do in emotionally charged situations such as waiting rooms. Suppressed anger leaks out in unexpected ways and may be manifested as poor time keeping, bullying, theft, and so on.

Stretching the miles

A social work manager found that one member of her team was making substantially bigger expenses claims than his colleagues. When this was investigated she found that the worker was angry and dissatisfied. He worked in an area of social deprivation and had many clients who failed to keep appointments and did not stick to agreed targets. He often made wasted journeys, and had taken to exaggerating his mileage claims as an angry response to his frustration.

Counselling helped him to find alternative ways of expressing his frustration. Because the problem was detected in good time, further escalation was avoided and a more serious level of disciplinary action was averted.

When stress becomes unmanageable and an employee is unsuccessful in finding ways to cope with the 'fight' or 'flight' response to adrenalin, she may resort to the 'freeze' response. This may result in a defensive paralysis or inactivity, symptoms of depression or numbing of the emotions. When this happens the carer turns into an automaton, just doing the job and not letting difficult feelings get in the way. This is an effective short-term strategy, but eventually her system will become overloaded and it will be impossible to keep all the emotion under control. Then a change in circumstances or a new event may release unexpected emotions. This is what happened to Joy.

Joie de vivre

Joy, a nurse who had pursued a professional career in nursing for over 20 years, attended the staff counselling service. She had become aware that she had no real zest for life, and did not experience the emotions of joy and ecstasy that she observed in others. She had a loving family but had not lived at home since starting her nurse training. Family visits were infrequent due to her professional commitments. She worried that there might be something wrong with her because she felt so lacking in emotion. As far as we could ascertain there had been no major traumas in her life, and other markers for depression were absent.

During the counselling process the picture gradually emerged that she hated hurting people. Her work had often involved performing procedures that were painful, such as changing dressings, giving injections and moving injured patients. She had developed a defence against emotion, especially pain. Her containment gave her a professional persona that enabled her to cope with work, but her other feelings were also suppressed, resulting in emotional disengagement. The defence extended into personal areas of her life.

Joy's emotional detachment was apparent to her counsellor, and gentle exploration enabled Joy to look at the way it affected her personal life. She started to practise being elated in appropriate situations, and was gradually able to expand her emotional repertoire. Creative use of her feelings also gave her more opportunity to process the stress of her working life.

Splitting

The psychological phenomenon of splitting may be viewed as another kind of denial. It arises from a tendency that some people have to see things in polarised terms such as good or bad, healthy or ill, functional or dysfunctional. Once this perception is in place, it is possible to ignore or split off the unwanted category. Health and social care workers are vulnerable to this process because of the nature of their work. Social workers represent a functioning welfare system, in contrast to their clients' often chaotic lifestyle. Doctors and nurses are usually healthy, in contrast to their sick patients.

In Chapter 1 the idea was explored that the decision to work in health or social care is sometimes based on a subconscious desire to remain healthy, or to avoid deprivation. In reality these polarisations are artificial. Social workers may be disorganised, and doctors and nurses sometimes become ill. One of the functions of staff support services is to help employees to recognise when their perceptions have become skewed. Stan (*see* page 69) had to recognise that he is not superhuman or above making mistakes – he is an ordinary human being doing a difficult job.

Splitting sometimes helps workers to cope with fear of distressing illness. Oncology is regarded as a highly stressful specialty. Often patients have to be given bad news. Cancer strikes fear into our hearts because sufferers may have to undergo surgery and unpleasant treatment, and in many cases the treatment is unsuccessful and the patient may die. Doctors and nurses find it hard to face cancer, too, but if they focus on the patients they avoid having to think about their own vulnerability. They tend to block out or split off their own fear of the disease.

Patients who are being investigated for possible malignant conditions are already anxious. They have to undergo a series of investigations and wait for the results to come back. The limbo state of not knowing is difficult to bear. I have heard many people say that they would rather know the worst than exist in the abyss of uncertainty. It usually falls to the doctor to give the bad news and offer treatment. Breaking bad news means confronting painful reality, and it is a neglected skill. Understandably some doctors try to avoid it while also recognising that doing it well can make a great difference to how the patient copes with the aftermath.

Why me?

Jose, a medical registrar, attended a training course on 'Breaking Bad News.' He worked in a department for chest diseases and many of the patients were being investigated for possible cancer of the lung. One of his duties was to take a weekly clinic where those patients who had completed their investigations were attending to be given their results. He found this clinic extremely stressful and felt that he spent the whole afternoon giving out bad news. Because he found it so difficult, he tried to do it as quickly as possible and messages were getting back to him that his approach was callous and unfeeling. He had been sent on the course to learn how to handle the breaking of bad news better.

During the group discussion it emerged that the clinic had several doctors, and some of the patients were being given good news, not bad. However, a selection process was going on, so that Jose was given many of the bad news cases. His colleagues had found a way to get more than their share of the good news cases, leaving him with a more stressful load. They had divided the caseload into good and bad, and distributed the work unfairly.

As well as learning how to handle the difficult job of giving bad news, Jose also learned that he needed to be more assertive about getting a fairer share of the workload. Other colleagues who found breaking bad news equally difficult were avoiding the problem and therefore saw no need to go on the course.

Projection

Sometimes, instead of suppression or denial, unwanted emotions are dealt with by projection on to another individual. The 'badness' is lodged with someone else. Often this person is already distant or separate in some way. She is unconsciously identified as a possible scapegoat.

An unhappy department

A group of counsellors often expressed dissatisfaction about their manager. Their work was difficult and stressful. Some of the clients made good progress, but not all of them. From time to time clients would miss appointments without notice, or seem to make unreasonable demands. The counsellors would feel frustrated and angry about this, but were unable to express their feelings to the clients who had caused the problems. Instead they became angry with the manager of the counselling agency, as though the administration was at fault.

The manager was not a counsellor and was seen as being more comfortable with accounts and computer printouts than with emotions. She sat in a separate office and did not communicate much with the other workers at the centre. The counsellors perceived themselves to be 'good', and anger may have been a difficult emotion for some of them to handle. They felt that no one valued what they did, and they thought that the manager should have been more attentive to their needs. At meetings the discussion often became focused on how unhelpful the manager was, and how she didn't run the centre effectively. In fact many counsellors expressed the opinion that the centre would run better without her!

A supervisor realised what was happening – that bad feelings were being projected on to the manager. When she encouraged the counsellors to focus on their own feelings of frustration, and to own some of their anger about their clients, the atmosphere improved. However, the underlying problem was ongoing, as it was an unavoidable aspect of the work that clients did not always do what was hoped. This supervisor made sure that the topic of anger remained high on the agenda for creative discussion.

In this case the manager was already set apart by being an administrator rather than a counsellor, by having a separate office, and by working with computers instead of people. Of course the centre could not cope without an administrator. In addition to the expected functions, she also acted as a container for 'bad' emotions. This case history shows how important it is for counsellors to have a supervisor who can take an overview and provide remedial action to restore balance. If this had not been the case, the manager's position might have become increasingly uncomfortable until she either chose to look for another job or was dismissed.

In order for projection to take place a recipient must be available. In the above example, the manager may have perceived antipathy from the counsellors and she might then have felt incompetent at her job, in which case transference of negative emotion has taken place. If her confidence had remained unaffected by the counsellors' negative behaviour, she would have resisted the transference. In the case of Kirsty (*see* page 13) the counsellor values the client's emotional needs, thus imparting a sense of worth to the client. Counsellors and other carers may unconsciously pick up anxiety from their clients. Clients and carers may be able to gain a sense of calm from a counsellor or manager who is able to keep their head in a crisis. These are all examples of transference.

Addiction

Misuse of drugs and alcohol is another defence strategy that is used to blot out or avoid dealing with stress, anxiety and vulnerability. Alcohol and recreational drugs are readily available and many people use them to unwind in social settings. When social lubrication becomes a habit and then a need, addiction becomes an additional problem. To make matters worse, health professionals can often find ways of accessing drugs that are meant for patients.

Johnson[3] proposes that the choice of medicine as a career is an adaptive response to a fragile sense of self and self-esteem, resulting in the development of a need for patients, emotional detachment and denial of vulnerability. These in turn predispose to depression, drug and alcohol abuse and suicide. The need to appear professional and able to cope with difficult situations makes it harder for doctors to admit to stress and difficult for them to ask for help.

Doctors have high standardised mortality rates for cirrhosis of the liver, accidents and suicide.[4] These events are markers for substance abuse. Medics commonly prescribe treatment for themselves rather than seeking medical attention in the same way as the rest of the population. When a doctor does this she is also hiding or denying her problems. Doctors, nurses, dentists and pharmacists often have access to drugs in the course of their work, so it is all too easy for them to become dependent on drugs or alcohol. Addicts have a remarkable ability to deceive themselves and others about their dependency.

The problem is often compounded by the collusion of colleagues, who are aware that there is a problem but do not feel able to challenge their peers. They may fear harming their colleague's career, or perhaps it reminds them of their own vulnerability. So they defend themselves as well as their colleagues by pretending that there isn't a problem. It is easier to bury one's head in the sand than to stir up trouble. Action may only be triggered when patients are put at risk. Estimates of the number of doctors affected by drug and alcohol addiction vary from denial that the problem exists to the sensational. The British Medical Association reports that the figure for doctors is probably similar to that for the general population,[5] but this still represents a serious problem. Help is available from the National Counselling Service for Sick Doctors and other medical agencies once the doctor has admitted that she needs to address the problem.

Dependency on drugs and alcohol is a paradigm for other addictions. Compulsive caring is a type of addiction to the intangible dynamic of needing to be needed. Addiction to food is similar in that it satisfies a craving but, as with other addictions, the satisfaction is short-lived and soon more is needed to satisfy the continuing desire. Hospital dining rooms used to be comfortable places where there was a plentiful supply of wholesome food for nurses and other staff. Working unsocial hours and living on the premises meant that the nurses' home was just that – a home from home, with food provided.

The pace of work has changed so much that it is often difficult for nurses to take proper meal breaks. It is now more common for them to grab a snack during a spare moment, without taking time out. Eating disorders easily develop when appetite and regular meals are ignored. The cravings of addiction are based on deep unmet needs for love and approval that in reality can never be met by drugs, alcohol, food or the needs of others. Often the sufferers sink even further into low self-esteem and self-hatred, compounding the problem and reinforcing the downward spiral. The dilemma for family, friends and colleagues is how to help them to get help. One of the maxims of addiction agencies is that if someone close to you is worried about your drinking, drug use or eating disorder, that means you have a problem. Another is that addicts must address their own addiction – no one else can do it for them.

Addicts have a tendency to collect codependents around them who allow them to carry on with their self-destructive behaviour. Codependents are often compulsive carers. Many a nurse is married to an alcoholic. Only when the codependents stop propping up, caring for and making excuses for the addict will she be able to make progress. When both dependent and codependent are ready to face the reality of their situation they can start to change their lives for the better.

Stresses that are likely to occur in the caring professions

The culture and management practices of health and social care work give rise to a range of stresses. These were explored in an organisational context in Chapters 2 and 3. Some tensions are inherent in health and social care work, while others could be alleviated by better management. Sources of stress include the following:

- lack of control over workload
- long-hours culture
- little opportunity for time out while at work
- limited opportunity to share emotional concerns
- problems that seem to have no solution
- constantly advancing knowledge
- organisations in the process of change
- financial restrictions
- inadequate administrative support
- dealing with death
- complaints from patients or clients
- violence and aggression from clients or patients.

When new or unexpected events occur in any of these categories, the additional stress may overwhelm the worker's ability to cope.

Lack of control over workload

The demand for health and social care seems to be endless. Current Government policy encourages people to expect higher standards of care. Increased longevity leads to an increase in care needs over a lifetime. Medical and social needs are often determined by emergencies, or by events that are beyond our control. There is a certain element of excitement or adrenalin buzz in providing emergency care. For some workers this enhances their job satisfaction. For others the constant worry of what will happen next, and how to find a bed for the next patient or an emergency foster carer for a vulnerable child, becomes exhausting. Sometimes the only way to manage this seems to be to change job or department, or to leave the profession. The latter option leads to wastage of skilled personnel and is demoralising for both individuals and organisations. Ruby (*see* page 34) found that a message book was one way to control her workload. Angela (*see* page 77) tried to avoid facing the packed waiting room, and the doctor in 'Work–life balance' (*see* below) was given direction about controlling his work–life balance by a more senior colleague.

Government targets may be imposed in ways that cause difficulty for workers. The case of 'Waiting and waiting' (*see* page 60) shows how pressure to meet seemingly impossible targets may have an adverse effect on patient care.

Although it is important to collect information, and accurate record keeping is vital, it often seems that paperwork takes up too much of carers' time. Many health and social care professionals are frustrated by the need to fill in statutory forms that have no direct benefit for the patient or client.

Long-hours culture

Sometimes working longer hours is the response of workers who are unable to control their workload. This may be a useful occasional strategy, but it is unsustainable as a regular solution. It exploits the good will of staff and increases stress. The boundary between work and personal life is threatened when there is no clear limit to the working day. Professional carers are often contracted to work unsocial hours. Although the nature of the job makes this unavoidable, it does place additional stress on family relationships. A supportive partner and family are recognised as important contributions to a worker's ability to cope with stress.[6] Damage to these relationships due to an inappropriate work–life balance has the knock-on effect of threatening a possible source of support.

The long-hours culture is a phenomenon that spreads through departments. If managers or role models set an example of working beyond contracted hours, junior staff may feel obliged to do the same. On the other hand, they may be instrumental in setting an example of a more appropriate work–life balance.

Work–life balance

A young doctor found without warning that he felt unable to face going to work. As he had young children he had made a conscious choice that he wanted to be involved in family life, and this meant marking time on the career ladder for the time being. He was referred to the staff counselling service by the Occupational Health department. His opening statement was 'I don't know what the matter is, but it might be to do with my mother's death last year.' He had found it difficult to separate the professional and personal aspects of his mother's hospitalisation, and could not stop analysing the clinical decisions made by her carers.

After her death he experienced feelings of guilt at not being able to do more for her. Logically he knew that the outcome was inevitable and all that could be done had been done. When trying to do his own work he had high professional standards and he always tried to do his best for his patients. This was coloured by saying to himself 'This patient is somebody's mother, husband or other loved one', which put extra pressure on him to do his best.

Despite his decision to focus on his family, he found it impossible to avoid being drawn into doing more than his basic job – for example, becoming a staff representative, lobbying for improvements and starting research projects. The shortcomings of the NHS became an increasing source of frustration for him.

This doctor's counsellor helped him to process some of the understandable grief about his mother's death, and also to have a clearer sense of boundaries. Over-identification with his patients had made it difficult for him to be objectively professional. The boundary between his personal life and his work was indistinct. Although he had made a conscious choice about his work–life balance, this was more difficult in practice than he anticipated. It is very hard not to be sucked in when the medical system is competitive and status driven. This young doctor was conditioned as a child to receive approval for academic success. In time he will perhaps learn to choose his own level of balance between intellectual recognition and family life according to his values rather than those of his parents.

The occupational health physician was more directive than the counsellor and forbade the doctor to take on any extra commitments. Psychologically the male physician provided a role model that emphasised approval of family values. Regular follow-up consultation was a condition of the young doctor's return to work. When a client wants to change established behaviour, follow-up provides an opportunity for ongoing reinforcement of the message.

This case history also demonstrates how the presenting symptom is rarely the whole story. Bereavement, work–life balance and childhood conditioning were all relevant to this case. When the counsellor or manager can tease these out there is hope for new understanding that will enable the worker to learn new coping strategies.

Little opportunity for time out at work

A constant state of alertness occurs when workers do not occasionally stop for a break. Eventually unrelieved stress leads to exhaustion, and a worker in this state may make mistakes and will not be able to work effectively. Taking regular breaks allows adrenalin levels to subside and stress levels to go down. The working environment in a hospital means that the workload is often very visible in the form of a ward or a waiting room full of patients. For a social worker it may be the bulging file of casework or the fact that the telephone never stops ringing that makes it seem impossible to stop working and take a break.

The waiting room

Angela is a skilled technician who works in an outpost department at a community hospital. There is never any let-up in her day because the waiting room is always full of people waiting for tests. Patients also spill over into the corridor, and sometimes there are not enough chairs for them to sit down. In the past, Angela asked for extra help from the main department, but there was rarely any available. She found it easier to cope if she stayed in the machine room and her assistant went to call the patients in. When she did not have to face all the waiting patients, she was better able to concentrate on her work.

However, things did not improve. The outpost department was enlarged to cope with extra demand, but Angela did not get any additional staff. It was only when she made a mistake that the situation changed. She was disciplined and was too distressed to go to work for several weeks. She spent days unable to do anything other than stare out of the window. At first she thought her whole career would come to an end.

The main department was forced to see how overloaded the laboratory had become when the replacement technician refused to work unless more assistance was provided.

Angela has returned to work, but she no longer works in the outpost department. She felt that her recovery was delayed because of the anger she felt about the lack of support, and also about her own inability to make her needs known. Counselling gave her permission to vent her anger, and also to learn to be more aware of her own needs. She developed assertiveness that enabled her to ask for and receive more support at work and in other areas of her life.

Limited opportunity to share emotional concerns

Increasing workload and a culture of not taking proper meal breaks, together with the loss of social space such as dining rooms, removes opportunities for informal contact with colleagues. It is harder to share emotional concerns when these opportunities are lost. Stan's story (*see* page 69) illustrates a culture of ignoring emotional distress that is common among healthcare workers and other carers. It comes from the previously explored concepts of denial and splitting. Stan felt that he must remain in control. Expressing vulnerability would seem to threaten his competence.

Joy (*see* page 71) also learned to keep her emotions under control at work, but this had a detrimental effect on her personal life.

Problems that seem to have no solution

Health and social care workers often have to deal with seemingly insoluble problems. They have to find a way of reconciling conflicting interests such as care and control. A professional carer's personal values may sometimes differ from the official guidelines that she has to put into practice.

Social deprivation has a habit of recurring down the generations, and social workers face a continuing cycle of needy clients. When a social worker sees the same problems in generation after generation of families she must sometimes wonder if her work makes much difference.

Children in care

This is a case from the family court. Sally was the social worker for a 15-year-old girl whose behaviour was out of control. She rarely went to school, and her foster mother often did not know where she was at night. The girl was staying in a squat and was using illegal drugs. Sally thought that it was likely she was involved in prostitution, but could not prove this.

When the girl had a baby, the court came to the conclusion that the baby should be taken into care for safety. Both Sally and her client were devastated by this, but for different reasons. The girl really wanted to try to be a mother to her child, but her chaotic lifestyle made this impossible. Sally knew that her client had also been taken into care as a small child and had had several foster carers, causing frequent disruption in her life. Would the same thing happen to this new baby? She had little faith that the system could do any better the second time around.

This scenario was a familiar one for Sally, who worked in a city-centre social services department. She continued in her job for a few years after qualifying as a social worker, but eventually she became worn down by the repetition of seemingly hopeless cases. At that point she decided to switch to temporary office work, where she felt she had no commitments and could walk away from the problems at the end of every day.

Seemingly insoluble problems are a daily reality for social workers and their colleagues in the health service. Caring for the sick is a never-ending job. Across the whole spectrum of illness the proportion of conditions that can be completely resolved is very small. Curable diseases take up relatively little time and effort. The huge mass of chronic health problems such as diabetes, heart disease, asthma, arthritis and cancer are treatable, but rarely curable. In the end the patient must learn to live with her illness and medical attendants can only help to stop things progressing quite so quickly. Most of the work is for people with chronic conditions that require ongoing treatment and monitoring. Often the patient's condition will gradually deteriorate however good the treatment is.

Patients are sometimes disappointed by their treatment or care. When a carer is unable to make a great deal of difference she is disappointed, too. Much dedicated care goes into trying to improve the quality of life for people with long-term illnesses. Complications will be prevented or postponed, but gradually things will get worse. This type of caring mostly takes place in primary care centres and care homes, and is very draining for carers and patients alike.

When patients do not get better, or they die, a worker who has chosen a career as a professional carer in order to make people better is constantly faced with failure. If she can gain a perspective that values partial success, this may help her to cope. Colleagues, managers and counsellors are all involved from time to time in reminding carers of the value of their work, even when success seems elusive.

Constantly advancing knowledge

Medical research gives hope of greater understanding of diseases and more effective treatment in the future. It may be intellectually rewarding for those involved, although there is often a great deal of tedious detailed work behind the scenes. Advancing knowledge means that patients can now be offered more treatments that give a hope of cure. These treatments can be invasive and traumatic in themselves, but if the end result is good such treatment will be worthwhile. For practitioners, advancing knowledge means that they always have more to learn – the journey to excellence never ends.

Specialised information is no longer limited to professionals, and patients can find out about their illness on the Internet. When patients become well informed in this way the doctor's superiority is challenged. One of the planks of the doctor's security is removed when she is no longer the sole source of specialist knowledge. The hierarchical relationship between doctors and patients is changing, so that now they are more likely to be engaged together in finding the best way forward. The responsibility of coping with illness is shared differently, giving the patient more control than before. A doctor may welcome this change in attitude if she can accept the loss of control involved.

Organisations in the process of change

As well as the changes that come from increasing knowledge, organisational change is a feature of health and social care, and was explored in Chapters 2 and 3. For many people working in this sector it creates a sense of insecurity, as there is no stability, and no time to consolidate new practices before yet more change is introduced. Change is often the extra stress that tips a carer who is just about coping with her work into overload and collapse. It may be the precipitating factor that leads a worker to seek help from support services. Managers need to be aware of the potential for change, including change for the better, to destabilise a department.

Financial restrictions

Increasing workload, advances in treatment and changes in management all result in increased costs. Financial resources for health and social care usually outstrip inflation, but the equation never seems to balance. As a result it often seems as if progress is inhibited by financial restrictions, and this causes frustration for health and social care workers. This is yet another aspect of the conflict between care and control that is such a feature of professional caring. Ongoing and unresolved conflict is stressful, due to the need to always be ready to adjust and make choices as to the best course of action. When the adrenalin cycle is fully charged, but release of stress is blocked, emotions may be released in an unpredictable way.

Making ends meet

Darren was referred to a staff support counsellor after he failed to report for work for two days without explanation. His work as a social worker for families with highly dependent children with special needs often took him away from his office, so for the first day his absence was assumed to be due to the fact that he was out visiting clients. On the second day his colleagues realised that he had not been seeing clients, so attempts were made to contact him. His manager quickly realised that Darren needed help.

When Darren started talking to his counsellor, he was unable to control his anger, shouting, swearing and storming round the room. After he had let off steam in this way he calmed down a little and was able to say more about what was troubling him. He had discovered that the budget for providing respite care for children in his caseload was fully spent, and he was unable to face the task of telling families that they would have no more respite until the new financial year. He knew how important this respite was in enabling these families to cope with ongoing heavy demands, and he dreaded being unable to help them.

Counselling could make no difference to the availability of funds, but Darren found it helpful to release his frustration in a safe atmosphere. His counsellor also helped him to rehearse what he could say to his clients to inform them of the shortfall, and to anticipate how he might respond to their anger at being let down by the system.

Inadequate administrative support

Professional carers need a range of ancillary workers to support their work. Sometimes the personnel who are not in direct contact with patients or clients are caught up in systemic problems. A secretary was sent for counselling because she had taken an excessive amount of sick leave. The departmental complement of secretaries had been reduced, she was unable to cope with her workload and she had inadequate support from her manager.

The mountain of work

Ruth was feeling overwhelmed by her work and had been asked to report to her manager to explain her high rate of sickness absence. This was the last straw for her and resulted in the manager recommending that she should use the staff counselling service. She was one of only two secretaries working for a large group of consultants. The agreed figure was five secretaries, although this had been reduced from a previous level of seven after a staff review. There were three unfilled vacancies.

Ruth felt unable to face the mounting pile of report typing that covered every available surface in her office. It had got to the stage where nothing could be found and urgent work was being delayed, to the detriment of patient care. She felt that if she protested she would incur further disciplinary action, and she feared that if she looked for another job she would not get a good reference.

In addition, she had taken on some heavy commitments to help her family.

The lack of administrative support for the whole department precipitated the collapse of Ruth's already stretched personal coping mechanism. She had learned to shoulder responsibility at an early age and saw herself as the only one who could deal with it. She had no sense that those in charge would help her or do anything to change the situation.

The organisational response to improve the output of the department had been to appoint another consultant, but this did not address the fact that the bottleneck in the system was at the point where reports were typed. It merely resulted in more reports and added to the problem. The vulnerable employee felt to blame for the failure of the whole system, just as she took on the responsibility for her family's problems.

When her coping strategy of taking sick leave was questioned, she experienced this as a disciplinary measure rather than as concern for her well-being. She felt that no one in her line management was taking her concerns seriously enough to make changes that would lift the block in the work process. The only other escape she could think of was to resign, but she was not confident of getting another job, and dreaded being unable to meet her family commitments.

Ruth's story illustrates the way in which damaging early experience sometimes causes people to repeat dysfunctional coping strategies. The resonance between her family system and her work system resulted in a dramatic worsening of her ability to cope. She also became the symptom carrier for a malfunctioning department. As is so often the case, the most junior or most vulnerable member of staff was the one to give way.

Systemically it is also worth noting that the solution proposed by the clinical director, a doctor, was to appoint an additional doctor. A consultant's salary would pay for three or four secretaries, and this would have made an immediate difference to the backlog of work. In fact the extra doctor created more work for the already overloaded secretaries, thus making the problem worse, not better.

Dealing with death

Fear of death was explored in Chapter 1. Healthcare workers cannot easily avoid the issue of death. In some specialties, such as cancer care and care of the elderly, death is always close at hand.

For staff working in oncology departments a high degree of optimism is necessary to carry the patients through the difficult treatments. Sometimes the treatment is unsuccessful or the side-effects may be worse than expected, or after a period of remission the cancer may recur. Doctors and nurses have to balance optimism and realism. They must be able to answer difficult questions from patients in a way that is appropriate for each individual. Great resilience is needed to cope with these ups and downs on a regular basis. Staff may become worn down by a series of treatment failures.

I was called upon to run a staff support group for an oncology ward that was experiencing a high level of stress. There had been a succession of young patients suffering from leukaemia or lymphoma, two of whom had recently died. The nature of the illnesses and the treatment meant that the patients had spent prolonged periods in hospital and the nurses had developed a very close relationship with them and their families. They had ministered to all their needs and carried out intimate care such as bathing and toileting, as well as intravenous and other drug treatment.

When after all this care the patients did not recover, some of the staff felt a sense of failure and a personal sense of bereavement. It is almost impossible to remain free from emotional involvement in this type of environment. These carers found it helpful to share their sense of loss and inadequacy in a protected group setting. Some carers find that they can only work in a highly stressed specialty for a limited period, and ask for rotation or transfer to a different ward in order to avoid burnout.

Sometimes it is hard to maintain a sense of perspective. I worked on a paediatric oncology ward at a time when I and several colleagues had young children. As most of our patients had serious illnesses, we worried about our own children too much. Every virus infection would seem like leukaemia, a swollen gland indicated Hodgkin's disease, or a fever must be septicaemia. There was a danger of our forgetting that most childhood ailments are trivial. We learned to support each other and sometimes to laugh at our foolishness. In this way we managed to keep our feet on the ground and our worries in perspective.

Pessimists do not find oncology congenial, as they tend to focus more on the negative aspects of the work. Optimists may sometimes find that their resilience is challenged when they are faced with repeated disappointment. Loss is always present in oncology. For the patient, the diagnosis brings fear of death or disfigurement. At the very least there will be invasive treatment and loss of freedom while the treatment is in progress. For the staff, repeated failure to meet their own expectations and those of users of the service can lead to disillusionment and burnout.

Loss crops up in all kinds of ways in health and social care. It constitutes an emotional milestone that frequently causes problems for staff. This is because it resonates with painful events in our own personal lives. People who choose to work in hospice and bereavement settings are especially vulnerable. I think it is fair to say that the relevant organisations are aware of this vulnerability and take care to provide the necessary support for staff. Maybe it is the carers themselves who sometimes forget and are taken unawares when their emotions are triggered. The bereavement process is a strange beast that is not easily tamed.

The bereavement counsellors Kubler-Ross and Kessler,[7] and also Worden,[8] have postulated a staged process through which those experiencing loss could process their grief and eventually move on. Structure is a helpful strategy for containment of overwhelming emotions. However, the process is rarely simple or orderly, and counsellors recognise that a bereaved individual often goes through an oscillating and interrupted journey to reach a stage where she can get on with her life. This does not necessarily mean getting over or forgetting her loss. It means a process of adjustment to her new status, or reframing of her place in the world.

Current experience of bereavement may recall grief from a previous unresolved loss. Care workers and others may be taken unawares when this happens.

Second childhood

Rose, a cleaner on a children's ward, came for bereavement counselling. Her husband had died suddenly six months previously. She was unable to carry on with her work because she kept crying for no apparent reason. The link with bereavement seemed to be the obvious cause of her distress. Rose talked freely about her deceased husband and enjoyed relating stories about their life together. She would often have imaginary conversations with him and would ask him 'up there' what he thought of events in her daily life. She seemed quite philosophical about his death.

Her early life had included many losses. She was abandoned as a baby and had been raised by nuns in an austere orphanage. She had had few personal possessions and no toys of her own. She recalled once being given a doll, but this had been confiscated on the pretext of needing a wash. It was never returned to her.

She felt unprepared for the outside world when she had to leave the orphanage at the age of 16, as she had no experience of ordinary home life. She did not know how to shop, cook or look after herself. Her husband had rescued her and gently introduced her to the ways of the world, and they were content in their own way.

As the counselling proceeded Rose felt better, but she still found it hard to return to work. Tears would return when she tried to do so. A shift occurred when the hospital chaplain asked her whether she was really happy in her job. He observed her in her working environment rather than in the counselling room and noticed that she became upset when one of the children in the ward was distressed. Maybe this touched a vulnerable spot for her inner child, with long-held grief from her early life.

She was baffled by the idea that this was the cause of her grief. It seemed irrelevant to her whether she was cleaning a children's ward or an adult ward. However, she agreed to try working on a different ward. The resulting improvement confirmed the chaplain's sense that it was childhood loss that was the problem, rather than the more recent death of her husband.

Sometimes grief may strike unexpectedly when a new event resonates with the past. Equally, staff in other situations that are not normally associated with loss can become very distressed when faced with death or terminal illness. They may have chosen to work to prevent death, or to work in a maternity ward where the atmosphere is mainly about birth, so they may be unprepared when unexpected death occurs.

When unusual or unpredictable events and changes are imposed on top of ongoing manageable stress, workers may be unable to cope. This is illustrated by several of the previous case histories. It is difficult to be prepared for problems that only occur occasionally. Laid-down procedures and policies may enable workers and managers to find out quickly what to do in unexpected circumstances.

Complaints

Professional carers set out to do their best to help people, so it is especially difficult when the recipients of care are not satisfied. Modern trends encourage complaints and litigation against professionals. It is increasingly important to remain aware of this possibility as an additional source of stress for health and social care workers.

The district nurse

Norma was referred for counselling when she had to face an enquiry after a patient's family filed a complaint about the way she had nursed their mother. The patient had been suffering from a terminal illness and was cared for in her own home by the local general practice team. Norma and her colleagues visited her daily and had agreed a treatment plan with the GP to relieve her pain. The plan was acceptable to the patient and her husband, but other members of the family were not happy with it. They had expressed their concern to Norma, but after consultation with the GP she continued as originally agreed.

After the patient died, Norma was accused of not providing the expected standard of care. For a professional with much experience this was a devastating accusation. It took her some time to regain her confidence after the complaint had been resolved.

Norma had followed an agreed treatment plan, and when this was questioned, she referred back to the plan and discussed it again with those involved. When a complaint was made, the primary care practice followed its complaints procedure. The process of investigation was aided by the fact that Norma and her colleagues had documented their actions and decisions at each stage. However, the effect on Norma's confidence was profound and disturbing. She was unable to return to work for several months.

This is also an example of the unexpected effects of loss and bereavement. The distress of family members at their relative's illness and death resulted in internal family disagreements being externalised to the carer. Their complaint was more about their own grief than about the carer's conduct. This type of complaint can be difficult to resolve, as it may not always be possible to unravel the source of the distress. Carers may often get caught up in anger and distress that rightfully belong to the patient or the recipient of care. People who are ill or vulnerable in other ways may be unable to look objectively at what is going on, and may then vent their anger on those who are trying to help.

The human instinct to seek to blame someone for what has gone wrong is very strong. This is still the case when what has gone wrong is due to natural events beyond our control. It takes great sensitivity to find out where there has been malpractice and deal with that appropriately while at the same time understanding the unresolved grief of the complainant.

When supporting the recipient of the complaint, a fine balance needs to be achieved. The worker will often have been suspended from duty pending enquiries, and may be forbidden to communicate with her peers or to speak to anyone about her case. A counsellor can provide understanding and behavioural strategies for stress management, but cannot take sides in the dispute. Unfortunately, the process of investigation may be prolonged, and serious loss of confidence can occur even if the eventual outcome is satisfactory.

The organisational aspects of complaints are explored in Chapter 3.

Violence and aggression from clients or patients

Care professionals work with patients and clients who are often angry or frightened. These feelings are understandable when the circumstances of a client's life seem to be in chaos. Part of the carer's job is to keep the situation under some degree of control. She has to manage her own feelings as well as trying to calm the client. Every so often this will be impossible and anger or violence will erupt. Staff have been injured or even murdered by their clients or patients. An NHS Staff Survey in 2004[9] reported that over a third of staff had experienced harassment, bullying or abuse at work during the previous year, and one-sixth had been subjected to physical violence. Mental health professionals, paramedics and ambulance technicians were most at risk of attack.

Safety begins with awareness – always being on the alert for possible danger and having a strategy in place to deal with it. If a worker is able to stay calm and resist the temptation to answer back, a risky situation is less likely to escalate. A little extra time allows her to summon support or take the distressed person to a place where she can express her feelings.

A serious safety incident leaves everyone involved feeling exhausted and vulnerable. If a worker does not have enough support from colleagues or her social network, extra help from a counsellor can help to release the tension. Individual or group debriefing sessions may be offered after a traumatic attack.

Personal attacks on carers cause psychological damage as well as physical injury. The balance of power between the carer and the recipient is challenged. If a carer is injured, she suddenly becomes the one in need of care instead of the giver of care – a brutal switch of roles. Workers who have been attacked sometimes find that they are unable to return to the same work when it seems that their fundamental values have been destroyed. The implied ingratitude of the attacker is too much to bear.

Sadly, aggression and bullying may also come from colleagues. Complaints about colleagues' professional conduct must be taken seriously and investigated. Both of these issues are sources of additional stress that may occur from time to time, so the relevant procedures and support services must be in place when the need arises (*see* Chapter 3 for more information about professional discipline).

Summary

For workers in health and social care, stress results from both personal constructs and organisational issues. Stress is a normal and necessary physiological response mediated by the adrenalin cycle. The purpose of this cycle is to maintain bodily function under a range of conditions and events. Most of the time this process of homeostasis takes place without conscious awareness. A sensation of stress only occurs when the usual range of stimulus is exceeded, or if stress continues over an extended timescale, thus disturbing the equilibrium.

The symptoms of stress are unpleasant and sometimes alarming. Chest discomfort, breathlessness and abdominal pain may mimic organic disease. At this stage many people are still able to recognise what is happening and take appropriate steps to reduce external stress and restore balance. They have a range of coping strategies that are brought into play when needed. If a worker is not aware of what is happening, or is unable to do anything to resolve the situation, ongoing stress may lead to emotional and physical breakdown and the syndrome of burnout.

The unconscious responses to stress include a range of psychological defence mechanisms. Denial, splitting, projection and substance abuse are familiar defences. They are linked to the personality traits that lead to the initial choice to work in the caring professions. In some cases they are amplified by training and by rewards received in the process of caring. These defences often help in the short term, but fail if the stress remains unresolved.

The culture of the organisations and the nature of the work of caring bring about certain stresses that are unavoidable. Often there is little or no control over workload, and workers are regularly faced with seemingly insoluble problems. The administration is constantly in a process of adaptation to new circumstances, and the knowledge base expands inexorably. There never seems to be enough money available, so unpalatable control is imposed from above. Workers must balance conflicting values of care and control, or square their personal morals with public policy. They often face death and disappointment, and their conscious and unconscious expectations of job satisfaction may be unfulfilled.

These ongoing processes provide a background level of stress that leaves little room for manoeuvre, so adverse events such as complaints, aggression or new administrative requirements are enough to tip the balance into loss of control. When normal coping mechanisms are insufficient, extra help is needed from managers and staff support services.

Awareness of the potential psychological vulnerability of care workers and the problems inherent in the work can enable managers and human resources staff to anticipate some of the issues. The case histories illustrate some of the ways in which workers are affected, and describe useful interventions. People choose to ask for help in various ways. Some people find it very difficult to ask for help, and delay doing so until the situation becomes unbearable. Others recognise that it is often best to nip things in the bud before too much damage has been done. Family, friends or religious leaders may give advice and support, or workers may approach their line manager, the occupational health service or a staff counselling service. Chapter 5 contains more information on how to provide professional support for those who work in the stressful occupations of health and social care.

References

1 Pines A and Aronsen E (1988) *Career Burnout.* Free Press, New York.
2 Fineman S (1985) *Social Work Stress and Intervention.* Gower Publishing, London.

3   Johnson WDK (1991) Predisposition to emotional distress and psychiatric illness among doctors: the role of unconscious and experiential factors. *Br J Med Psychol.* **64:** 317–29.

4   British Medical Association (1993) *Report on the Morbidity and Mortality of the Medical Profession.* British Medical Association, London.

5   Coombes R (2005) Shaken and stirred? *BMJ.* **330:** 1513.

6   Greenwood A (1997) Stress and the EAP counsellor. In: M Carroll and M Walton (eds) *Handbook of Counselling in Organisations.* Sage, London.

7   Kubler-Ross E and Kessler D (2005) *On Grief and Grieving: finding the meaning of grief through the five stages of loss.* Simon and Schuster, London.

8   Worden W (2003) *Grief Counselling and Grief Therapy* (3e). Routledge, Hove.

9   Commission for Healthcare Audit and Inspection (2005) *NHS Staff Survey 2004.* Commission for Healthcare Audit and Inspection, London.

Chapter 5

Support services

Introduction

The psychological motivation of professional carers working in health and social care, and the culture of the organisations in which they operate, provide fertile ground for work-related stress. When we do not pay attention to the fact that professional caring is a stressful occupation, there is a risk of damage to the emotional and physical health of employees. If this occurs, the employing organisations suffer from inefficiency, unsafe practices, and failure to meet the needs of patients and clients.

This chapter explores recent evidence that identifies the need for staff support in health and social care, and its potential benefits. Recommendations for provision of staff counselling are laid down in publications by the Health and Safety Executive and the Royal College of Nursing. I shall focus on the range of support services available, the value of counselling interventions to the emotional health of professional care workers, and the dilemmas encountered by counsellors and managers at the interface of the interests of employer and employee. Case histories further illustrate possible conflicts of interest.

Counsellors in workplace settings work with professional carers as clients, but they also have a responsibility to the employing organisation. This reminds us that systemic processes are an important aspect of work-related counselling. Supervision is an essential part of the counselling process, as it helps counsellors to make use of parallel process to understand what may be happening to their client in the workplace. I shall consider the unconscious processes that take place in the supervision system and link them to case histories in previous chapters.

The purpose of providing support for professional carers is to enable them to cope with stress, gain personal satisfaction from their work and therefore do a better job. The organisations that provide health and social care services, and the end users – the general public – also benefit from staff support services.

Why do we need support services?

The 2004 NHS Staff Survey conducted by the Healthcare Commission[1] showed that 40% of healthcare staff reported experiencing work-related stress during the previous year. A third of NHS staff in this survey agreed or strongly agreed that they often thought of leaving their job. A high rate of psychological morbidity was documented by Borrill et al. in a survey of staff at two NHS trusts.[2] In this survey, 28% of staff reported symptoms indicating mild or moderate mental illness. A survey by Caplan[3] of hospital consultants, general practitioners and senior health service managers indicated higher than expected levels of stress, anxiety and depression. In total, 47% scored high levels of stress, and managers were as likely to be stressed as doctors.

Less information is available about social workers. Collings and Murray[4] linked high levels of stress and dissatisfaction in social workers to high workload, pressure to complete paperwork, having no answers to specific client problems, and unsatisfactory supervision arrangements. Social workers who received little social or personal support were more stressed than those who had close family and peer support. Society's poor perception of social workers was perceived to be an additional factor causing stress.

A more recent survey by Huxley *et al.*[5] of mental health social workers showed that 47% had stress levels indicating a potential psychological disorder, and unfilled vacancies and poor staff retention were identified as causing significant extra stress. Vacant posts cause an additional burden for existing staff, who have to cover for absent colleagues in order to fulfil statutory requirements.

The *Working Well Survey* by the Royal College of Nursing demonstrated a clear link between poor psychological health and increased sickness absence.[6] Staff who were experiencing significant levels of psychological distress reported twice the mean level of sickness absence of their other colleagues. There has been no similar survey of social workers, but informal reports indicate that stress, dissatisfaction and absenteeism are also prevalent in this sector.

The human and organisational cost of work-related stress is unacceptably high, and employers now recognise that they should take care of their workers' welfare. The NHS Executive has made a commitment to reduce sickness absence and violence against staff,[7] and has produced a comprehensive guide to providing staff counselling in NHS settings.[8]

Good management practices are included in the NHS Executive recommendations for ensuring a healthy and effective workforce in the NHS. Managers and human resources personnel are also aware that staff support services are an important fringe benefit, and recognise that if staff feel cared for they are likely to be happier and more productive. Managers have an important role in encouraging members of staff who are experiencing psychological distress to seek help, because they may be a danger to themselves and their colleagues, patients and clients if they continue to work when unfit to do so.

Employers, including the NHS and local government authorities, have a legal duty to look after the safety and welfare of their workforce as set out in the Health and Safety at Work Act 1974. If they do not do so, and an employee's health is damaged, costly litigation may follow.[9] The expense of providing staff support can be justified on financial as well as humanitarian grounds. A systematic review by McLeod[10] found that counselling interventions are effective in alleviating many of the symptoms of anxiety, stress and depression. Sickness absence rates were reduced by 25–30% in clients who received counselling. The NHS Executive paper[8] contains case studies that demonstrate the cost-effectiveness of staff counselling services.

Professional carers expect that they will themselves be cared for when they work in a caring environment. This is not always explicit, but it is often cited as a cause of dissatisfaction when carers consult support agencies. The provision of staff support services gives workers a sense that they are valued, and signals that an organisation does have concern for the welfare of its staff. Even those who do not use the service gain confidence from knowing that it is available should they ever need it.

What support is available?

When a professional carer seeks help for stress, it is likely that she will already have made use of personal coping strategies and will have drawn on the support of friends and family. Sometimes it may not be possible or appropriate to do this. She may choose to get help, or she may be referred by a manager or occupational health officer.

The range of support available for professional carers reflects the fact that decisions about staff support are often made at local level, by NHS trusts, local government authorities and charities. Decisions reflect the size of the organisation and the perceived needs of the workers. Large organisations may find it cost-effective to have an independent scheme, while others may choose to purchase support services from a larger national or local provider.

Informal support

The majority of workers in health and social care who experience stress at work will have personal coping strategies and support from peers, friends or family that enable them to retain their resilience. The concept of stress as a normal and often benign physiological process mediated by the adrenalin system was explored in Chapter 4. Professional carers have become so busy that there is little opportunity to take a break, and there are few opportunities to share emotional concerns. When there is no time to reflect, self-awareness of stress is reduced.

Many professional carers feel that they work in isolation despite being in a large organisation. I worked for a time in a large London teaching hospital where there were hundreds of people walking through the corridors at all times of day. I only interacted with a small number of people in my immediate department, and I felt no sense of connection with the wider organisation. Nurses and care workers in the community often use their car as an office, and may have infrequent contact with colleagues back at base. Consequently they suffer a sense of isolation and lack of support. Human beings want a sense of belonging and a sense of being valued as individuals. Workers need to feel that somebody cares about their work and existence. When these values are eroded by organisational culture, it becomes necessary to put something in place to restore the balance.

Often people are able to do this for themselves and create their own opportunities for personal renewal. This may be as simple as talking things over with a partner, friend or colleague, or taking part in a recreational activity. This kind of release works well as a safety valve for regularly letting off the pressure so that stress and anxieties do not build up to overwhelming levels. It does depend on the existence of a close personal network of people who can be trusted to understand and also to respect confidentiality. It is worse than useless to confide in a friend and later find that the whole department knows about the problem. There is also an implicit expectation that the process will operate reciprocally. You will listen to your friend's problems if she listens to yours. This is not always possible, and the friendship may suffer under the strain.

Carers are often empathic towards their colleagues, and spontaneously offer support or suggest taking time out if this seems necessary. For many professional carers a mutually supportive relationship with colleagues enables them to keep going, and to retain a sense of proportion when work seems overwhelming.

Successful carers often seem to develop a personal 'toolkit for survival' that consists of self-awareness, stress-releasing activities and peer support.

Management responsibility

Managers give informal support, but also need to be aware of when to be more directive. A manager who is worried that a member of staff is becoming stressed at work may have to take formal steps to help her. When informal support is not enough, the manager may suggest a referral to occupational health services or a staff counselling service. A worker may not want to share personal issues with her manager, and it is sometimes inappropriate to do so. She may prefer to consult her usual general practitioner, especially if she has a good relationship with them already. Workers may seek a medical consultation for physical symptoms such as backache, or recurrent infections, which are sometimes a result of stress.

Managers have a vital role in ensuring that the working environment is safe and appropriate, and that systems are in place to respond to individual concerns. When there is a climate of trust, and good practice is valued, workers are able to freely express their concerns and work-related stress is less likely to become a problem. When managers promote a culture of learning from experience, problems and crises become opportunities for growth. Organisational learning, like individual personal development, is a lifelong process.

Although counsellors are trained to be alert for transference and counter-transference, managers may not always be aware of these non-verbal psychological processes.[11] Managers are responsible for the workers in their team, and this inevitably affects their interactions. At different times a manager gives instructions, oversees work done by others and directs compliance with official procedures. Managers and colleagues cooperate to achieve desired goals.

An employee may see her manager as a parental figure, or as a mentor, and consequently positive or negative feelings may be aroused. A parent may be nurturing, critical or punitive in different circumstances, and these attributes also occur in the employee–manager relationship. If a worker has experienced a nurturing relationship with her parents, she is likely to expect this type of response from her manager. Similarly, if her parents were always critical, she may anticipate that her manager is also likely to be critical. These unconscious expectations (transference) may colour the interactions between employee and manager before any relationship has been established. Equally, a manager's previous experience influences her management style, and she may unconsciously respond to situations in ways that reflect her personal conditioning. This is known as counter-transference.

Not good enough

Social workers face a tide of needy clients that sometimes seems overwhelming. James works with vulnerable young adults, and often feels that the resources for his clients are inadequate. He has a sense of personal inadequacy about being unable to do more for the young people who are struggling to find their feet in the adult world after growing up in care. James recognises that he empathises with his clients because of his personal experience during childhood. His father was always urging him to do better at school. He hoped that James would make the best of his abilities, but the effect on his son was to make him feel that he was never good enough. Encouragement was not reinforced by praise for his achievements, and James still feels that he is not good enough.

He dreads meetings with his manager because he fears that his inadequacy will be exposed. James' manager is an experienced social worker who is well aware of the difficulties that James faces in his work, so he gives positive feedback about what James is doing for his clients. To his surprise, James seems not to hear him and reacts as if he is being criticised. Neither of them knows how to deal with this misunderstanding, so they pretend that nothing untoward is happening.

Afterwards the manager reflects and decides to keep a closer eye on James, taking opportunities to give him informal encouragement. In due course, James gains confidence and is able to accept praise. He becomes happier and more effective in his work, learning that senior male colleagues are not necessarily like his father. His manager used his experience to recognise how to nurture young talent in a way that is not threatening.

Managers who understand how previous life experience can affect unconscious processes in the workplace are more effective in their interactions with their colleagues. Sometimes it is necessary to stand back and ask the following questions: 'What is happening? What other factors are coming into play? Why am I getting this response?' A good manager knows when to encourage, when to delegate responsibility and when to discipline. For some, this ability is acquired naturally. Appropriate training also helps managers to develop these skills.

In my experience, health and social care organisations are good at encouraging career development, and offer a nurturing environment to workers who want to improve, but formal management training is often lacking. Workers who perform well at their job are sometimes promoted to managerial positions for which they have no proper training. The transition from worker to manager represents a significant shift, and is one aspect of the stress caused by organisational change that was explored in Chapter 2. If a professional carer becomes a manager, the move from a caring role to a controlling role may not be a comfortable transition. Social workers, nurses and counsellors may all find that career progression involves this change in emphasis.

Professional carers want to look after people. They often struggle with the need for control. Time and resources are limited, but needs seem to be endless. A manager's role often involves imposing control while at the same time maintaining a caring environment for both workers and patients or clients. Managers who have previously been carers may find it more difficult than they had expected to make the transition from being principally carers to being in control of budgets, staff and employment issues. They must balance care and control in order to achieve an effective service.

Jackie in transition

Jackie is a home care worker who is very dedicated to her job as a personal carer for patients with severe long-term disabilities. She has developed health problems, and after a significant amount of sick leave she has realised that she cannot offer the level of care that is necessary to meet her clients' needs. She has a meeting with her manager and her human resources representative to discuss her future employment, and together they explore ideas for a solution.

Jackie is realistic about her health but does not want to give up work. She likes the idea of using her experience to become an assessor for client care packages, and is enthusiastic about finding out what further training she might need for this role. She confides her doubts to her counsellor. With this change, Jackie would miss the opportunity she now has to build up a relationship with her clients. She also thinks that she might want too much for the clients she assesses: ' I would want them to have everything, and sometimes that can't be done.'

She is starting to recognise that a job change might entail a shift in her personal philosophy, and is not sure that she is ready to take this step. She has not previously considered the ambivalence of care and control. She is also facing the ambivalence of her own change of status from healthy to needy. In future she may be the recipient of care, instead of a giver of care.

Ambivalence emerged during the process of counselling that was initially directed at enabling Jackie to return to work. This case history shows how unexpected unconscious issues may arise in counselling. Skilled and experienced counsellors are alert for new disclosures, and have to judge whether any new issues can be properly dealt with in short-term counselling.

In the case histories of both Jackie and James, managers were involved in helping workers to cope with emotional difficulties. Awareness and sensitivity on the part of the managers helped the process of adjustment. It may be that they had received training in counselling skills, enabling them to be empathic and open to the possibility of unconscious processes. However, these managers also realised that both of these workers could benefit from sessions with a trained counsellor. Counselling skills are very useful for managers and professional carers, but cannot replace the experience and objectivity of a counsellor.

Some parts of the health and social care professions have a separate management training hierarchy. This has the advantage of clearly distinguishing between care and control roles, but may carry the danger that managers are unaware of the stress of caring. They may then fail to recognise the emotional needs of the staff whom they manage.

Doctors have a very loose managerial structure, so their welfare at work may be overlooked. It is not safe to assume that doctors will be adequately aware of their own needs, and peers may feel inhibited about giving advice on stress when this may be perceived as a criticism. Despite having high stress levels, doctors are reluctant to ask for help and are infrequent users of support services.

The traditional hierarchy in medicine perpetuates a paternalistic system. If a consultant is nurturing and appropriately challenging, trainee doctors benefit, but there are many instances of damage to the psychological health of young doctors when consultants have been critical or dismissive. Supervision and mentoring of trainee doctors are directed at achieving training goals, and their emotional needs may be neglected. When doctors do have access to staff counselling services, they often find it difficult to attend regular appointments. Clinical commitments such as ward rounds, operating lists and clinics, together with the on-call bleeper, give them limited control over their time. Counsellors do try to be flexible, and doctors can find the necessary time when they accept the benefit of counselling. Unfortunately, the process of stress and burnout may be far advanced by the time this happens.

A counsellor who was providing help for patients on an oncology ward met with scepticism from the doctors on the ward. However, when one of the doctors had personal experience of the devastation of a cancer diagnosis and received counselling for this, her attitude changed and she spread the word among her colleagues about the benefits of counselling. Managers and senior professional carers must remember to look after their own emotional needs as well as those of their juniors. They have the same rights to access support services as other staff, and should be equally sure that their confidentiality will be respected.

Professional bodies and unions

The British Medical Association (BMA) regularly publishes papers and editorials about stress, to help doctors to become more aware of their vulnerability. BMA members have access to a telephone counselling service from a national Employee Assistance Programme (EAP) provider. Some local healthcare trusts also provide support services specifically for doctors. Doctors in practice are required to have professional indemnity insurance, and this would include the support of legal representation for employment issues as well as for complaints from patients.

The Royal College of Nursing has a counselling service for members, provides legal advice and representation on employment matters, and has produced a comprehensive range of publications giving guidance on stress and welfare at work in the 'Working Well' series.

The professional body for social workers is the British Association of Social Workers. This association provides legal advice, representation and assistance with regard to employment issues. It does not provide a counselling service, as it expects employing organisations to do this. Thus, unlike nurses and doctors, social workers do not have a dedicated source of counselling linked to their specific issues. Local authority employers have such a wide range of workers that the needs of carers, as distinct from those of other workers, may not be adequately catered for. Social workers in voluntary settings rely on the support provided by each individual charity.

Workers in professions allied to medicine, and those in administrative or other supporting roles may belong to other unions. UNISON provides listening and support for debt, legal advice and representation on employment matters, and other benefits including holiday breaks, but does not have a counselling service for members. Amicus provides legal advice on employment matters, stress management and guidelines on health and safety matters, but does not offer a counselling service.

The British Association for Counselling and Psychotherapy (BACP) is an accrediting body, and its journals provide a forum for exploring issues relating to counsellors' needs for self-awareness and support. It also publishes guidance on ethics and sound practice. BACP insists on regular supervision for registered practising counsellors. In addition, there is a requirement for professional indemnity insurance. This usually also covers legal costs for practice-related litigation. Counsellors are expected to undergo personal therapy as part of their training, and are recommended to continue with this as an additional element of self-care. Counsellors are professional carers who try to do for themselves what they recommend others to do – in other words, look after their own emotional and physical health.

Occupational health services

To provide for the welfare and safety of workers, occupational health departments offer both preventive and responsive services. Prevention includes pre-employment medicals, immunisations, and recommending healthy practices in the workplace. Employees may need help in managing ongoing medical conditions while at work, or when returning to work after a period of absence due to ill health. Recurrent absence may be investigated in case a worker's health is being damaged by her working conditions. The occupational health physician will usually be able to help an employee to negotiate with her manager for a staged return to work if this is needed. If illness is serious or prolonged, the occupational health physician may have to decide whether it is possible for the employee to return to work. Retirement on the grounds of ill health or alternatively a change of job may be recommended.

Stress is often manifested as physical symptoms, so the occupational health department may be the first port of call for a distressed worker. Health professionals may be more willing to consult about health-related symptoms than about emotional distress, because the language and culture of health are familiar to them. Doctors and nurses in occupational health departments need to be aware of the possibility of underlying stress when workers present with physical symptoms, especially if these are recurrent.

A stressed carer may ask for counselling, or the occupational health physician or general practitioner may refer her to a counsellor, a clinical psychologist or a psychiatrist, according to their assessment of the problem. Provision should be made for employees to self-refer directly to a counselling service. Clinical psychologists are likely to offer cognitive–behavioural therapy (CBT) directed at stress management or the treatment of symptoms of panic and anxiety. CBT is an effective intervention for these.[12] Severe depression and mental disturbance cannot usually be effectively treated by short-term counselling. It is important to recognise the limitations of counselling, so that appropriate referral can be made for longer-term treatment.

It is not always clear to employees whether an occupational health service is for the benefit of the organisation or the employee. For this reason, many workers are afraid to ask for help in case they are labelled as 'unfit', and they are concerned that this may affect their prospects of promotion. The involvement of occupational health services in the investigation of absence from work is often seen as punitive. When an emotional crisis is clearly affecting performance at work, an employee may be asked to seek counselling or may be sent to the counselling service. I have occasionally had clients brought to counselling by managers or colleagues. However, counsellors may have difficulty in building a therapeutic relationship with a client who has been referred for counselling against their will. It is usually best if clients choose to get help for themselves. They are then more likely to be committed to the process.

A statistic

Jenny was referred to occupational health when she had been off work for 3 months due to a succession of infections and minor operations. In discussion with her manager she had gained the impression that the manager was more concerned about meeting targets to reduce absenteeism than about Jenny's health. The occupational health counsellor had to help Jenny to process her anger about this before any therapeutic trust could be established. A phased return to work was agreed with her manager, and Jenny said later that this was helpful in enabling her to face the prospect of returning to work.

Jenny was in danger of losing confidence in her ability to return to work, and the intervention of a counsellor helped her to regain her emotional strength. When she started the phased return, her self-esteem visibly improved, and Jenny admitted that counselling had been 'good for her', despite her initial scepticism about it.

Occupational health departments are concerned about the interests of both employees and employing organisations. These usually coincide, as both benefit from a healthy working environment and a healthy workforce.

Counselling services often come under the umbrella of an occupational health department, but in most cases they are operated as a self-contained unit. This ensures confidentiality and separation of any counselling records from medical notes. For administrative convenience, occupational health departments may provide line management, premises and administrative services for such counselling units. Counselling may be financed by occupational health, human resources or departmental budgets, according to local arrangements.

Counselling

Counselling is a professional therapeutic intervention that aims to help a client to explore and understand her emotional reactions. She can then, if she wishes, make informed choices to resolve emotional and behavioural problems. Counselling is usually a one-to-one activity, or a couple may attend together to explore relationship problems with a counsellor. There is a distinction between counselling and counselling skills. Many people possess a natural ability to listen empathically and non-judgementally, while others learn to do this by experience, or undergo counselling skills training. These are valuable traits, but they stop short of the knowledge and experience of an accredited counsellor. Sometimes people who seek counselling do so because they fear overburdening their friends with their problems. Friendly support may carry an assumption of reciprocal sympathy. Counselling has the advantage that it focuses on the needs of the client. The counsellor listens to the client, but the client does not have to hear any of the counsellor's problems in return.

Group counselling

When a group or department has been collectively affected by a traumatic event or a stressful period, group counselling may be requested or offered. A disturbing event may affect several people, or organisational changes may affect a whole department. Sometimes ongoing stress is unavoidable. For example, it may be helpful to provide regular staff support group sessions for mental health units, intensive-care wards, neonatal units, hospices or human immunodeficiency virus (HIV) treatment units. Sometimes stress management or assertiveness skills training are provided as group activities for staff or clients. Group counselling may provide an opportunity for a care worker to venture into the arena of counselling when she does not want to face the spotlight alone. Individual counselling should always be available as well as group counselling. As with any counselling, the process may throw up unexpected emotions, and workers may need additional help for these situations in one-to-one counselling.

A group may be led by a counsellor or a clinical psychologist with appropriate experience. When a group is formed, the purpose and membership of the group should be defined, and explicit boundaries of confidentiality must be established. The group leader has the task of ensuring the safety of the group for its members, and also of keeping the group focused on its purpose. The dynamics of a group are different from those of individual counselling. The power of being part of a group may allow collective blaming of the organisation or other individuals, and attention may be diverted from addressing the real problem. A skilled facilitator will be aware of this and will help to keep the group focused on the task in hand.

Employee Assistance Programmes

Many employers choose to contract out Employee Assistance Programmes (EAPs). There are a number of national and international services that provide a telephone helpline, face-to-face counselling, legal advice and sometimes training and management support services for employees. In some schemes, family members are also entitled to use the service. Employees are usually given information about support services in a welcome pack when they join the employing organisation, and may then forget all about it. They may have to be reminded about the existence of these services when the need arises. It is useful to have information about support services on display in appropriate places, and to publicise the EAP from time to time.

The first contact between client and counsellor is usually made by telephone. An assessment of the problem may be made over the telephone or in a face-to-face interview. Most EAPs aim to offer access to a counsellor by telephone during working hours, and sometimes a 24-hour service is offered. Helpful intervention for acute stress can be provided in this way. The counsellor who answers the helpline will make an assessment of the problem presented by the client, and can often provide telephone counselling there and then. Follow-up appointments for telephone counselling may be offered on a regular basis, or if the assessment shows that face-to-face counselling is more appropriate, arrangements are made for this. A database of associate counsellors around the country enables the EAP provider to match the client with a counsellor with relevant experience in a convenient location.

When counselling is provided in this way, an employee contacts the EAP directly, and should not need to inform her manager or anyone else. She may be advised by her manager, colleagues or occupational health practitioner to use the service, but it should be the employee's decision to do so. This arrangement is more likely to ensure confidentiality. Normally any counselling notes remain with the EAP and are not disclosed to the employer. There is no direct contact between the counsellor and the employing organisation – in fact the counsellor may not know who the employer is. The EAP may feed back statistical information to employers about the use of the service. The employer pays the EAP for the service provided, and the EAP pays the counsellors, again preserving confidentiality. The client does not pay directly for her counselling.

Some EAPs include a management consultancy service that aims to address any systemic organisational issues that are identified. For reasons of confidentiality, this would not be linked to specific clients. Clinical supervision and consultancy are provided by the EAP to counsellors as needed to support casework, but counsellors are required to have their own supervision and insurance arrangements.

A large EAP may be able to provide a more comprehensive service than an occupational health department. A 24-hour telephone helpline provides immediate support at times of crisis. Telephone counselling can be used to support clients until they are able to access face-to-face counselling or other services. EAP counselling is usually limited to a maximum of eight sessions. It is therefore important that EAP counsellors are experienced in short-term focused counselling. If longer-term counselling or therapy is needed, clients are referred to other sources of help – for example, via their general practitioner or a psychotherapist. Employers are unlikely to provide open-ended psychotherapy.

In some circumstances EAP counselling sessions are conducted by telephone. Employees who work irregular or unsocial hours may prefer telephone counselling. The BMA has a contract for telephone counselling for its members, on the grounds that doctors are too busy to attend appointments for face-to-face counselling. This may be one of the causes of their stress. It is possible that this restricted service provision colludes with doctors' tendency to deny having personal problems.

When a counsellor is exploring what is troubling a client, her initial assessment includes what is happening at work, and whether or not the counselling is for an EAP. She also needs to consider what else is going on in the employee's life that may resonate with their stress at work. Distressed workers can expect that counselling will help with a range of personal, health or work stresses with different degrees of severity.

Many workers try to keep their work life and home life separate. However, personal and work-related stress are interdependent. If an employee is overloaded at work, she will be too tired and stressed to cope with pressure at home, and vice versa. Boundary confusion occurs when events in the workplace spill over and become blurred with other areas of personal life. Stressful events in the present sometimes resonate with emotions from the past, resulting in unexpected fallout. A counsellor may be able to help a client to see that what is going on in one system mirrors events in another system, or that emotions belonging to one system are being projected on to another. Systems aspects of work-related stress were explored in Chapter 2.

A client may insist that she is looking for coping strategies that are relevant to her present problems. She may be reluctant to delve into the past, thinking that this is not relevant, and possibly fearing that forgotten traumas will be uncovered. However, some understanding of previous history often helps a client to make changes in her emotional reactions. She is more likely to gain lasting benefit if this happens. Teaching coping strategies alone may run the risk of restoring a client's equilibrium so that she can return to the same stressful scenario that caused the problem in the first place. If this happens, the client will probably relapse and may suffer further emotional harm.

The best results are obtained when a client is able to make a significant shift in her attitude, and at the same time changes occur in the organisational system. It is rare for problems to be caused solely by either the client or the organisation, although attempts may be made to blame one side or the other. A person-centred counsellor may easily be drawn into colluding with her client in blaming the job, the manager or the whole organisation for the client's problems. This is fruitless, as the client has little or no power to change the system, and she becomes diverted from the task of making her own changes. If a client is seen to be taking steps to help herself, her manager and colleagues may respond by considering systemic changes, as in Ruby's case (*see* page 34).

When counselling is provided by an employer, there is always the possibility of a conflict of interest in the triangular relationship between the employer, the client and the counsellor (*see* 'A statistic' on page 97 and 'Contracts in workplace counselling' on page 39). Although an employer or manager may be concerned about a worker's well-being, they will want her to be at work and functioning effectively as soon as possible. The counsellor may find herself in an uncomfortable position, pulled between the interests of her client and those of the employing organisation. However, a workplace counsellor is in a position to take an overview and to see the possibility of systemic dynamics in the relationship between her client and the employing organisation.

A dutiful daughter

Celia, an administrator, managed successfully to continue to do her job while looking after her elderly mother, whose health deteriorated over many years. Celia was also under considerable pressure at work because of departmental reorganisation.

Her mother later died, and this was the point at which all her coping ability deserted her and she took time off work with stress. To begin with neither Celia nor her doctor recognised the scale of the problem, and short-term absence gradually became long term. At this point she was referred for counselling. She had kept her emotions at bay for so long that, once she let go, there was a huge amount of reparation to be made.

The manager was clear about her expectation that counselling would expedite Celia's return to work. Understandably, in this case, the employer needed to know whether Celia would be able to return to work, and for how long they would have to provide locum cover. However, Celia needed more time to regain her strength and to rebalance her life. She found enquiries from the human resources department about her progress intrusive and threatening, and responded by withholding information. The counsellor also received requests for progress reports.

Information about a client's fitness for work should come from a consultation between the client and her GP or occupational health physician. If the counsellor is expected to provide this information, the safety of the counselling will be compromised. Therapy will not be effective if the client cannot trust her counsellor. In this example, the counsellor explored with her client what action should be taken. The client decided to be more open with her manager about the reasons for her delayed return to work. After further discussion with the occupational health physician, a plan for phased return was agreed.

In-house EAP schemes

In-house EAP schemes are clearly linked to the employing organisation that they serve, and may provide a service that is tailored to the specific needs of that organisation. Hospital EAPs are a case in point, where the needs of health workers are different from, say, those of engineering workers or retail staff. In-house schemes are usually sited on or near the workplace premises. Administration and counselling take place on the organisation's premises, and in some organisations counselling may also take place at associate counsellors' consulting rooms.

In-house EAP counsellors may be paid a salary, but more often they are paid on a client-by-client basis by the employing organisation. If counsellors are paid a salary, there may be confusion about pay scales. There is no clearly established pay scale for counsellors, and different organisations use different parameters to set counsellors' pay. Sometimes a nursing pay scale is used. (Many counsellors have previously worked as nurses.) In other cases, clinical psychology or occupational therapy pay scales may provide the baseline. This issue is currently under review for counsellors in healthcare settings, with the 'Agenda for Change' initiative to standardise pay scales across the NHS.

On-site counselling has some advantages for employees. It is less time consuming for them if they merely have to walk to another part of the site rather than having to travel to another unfamiliar location using public transport or spend time finding a parking space. Often a client can take an hour out of her working day without disruption, whereas travelling elsewhere would take a minimum of two hours for a one-hour counselling session.

On the other hand, confidentiality may be more difficult to secure than when the EAP is a separate organisation. The location of the counselling service may mean that passers-by can see clients going into the EAP office. Although the counsellors take great care to keep records in a confidential system, it is more difficult to convince clients that their confidentiality will be respected when the records are on site.

Contract with an EAP in a related organisation

A small organisation – for example, a private care home – will not have a large enough number of employees to sustain a counselling service of its own. A service set up by one organisation may utilise the economy of scale by contracting to provide services to other local employers. For example, a hospital EAP could contract to provide counselling to a neighbouring primary care trust, local government organisation or private care homes.

Private health insurance

Organisations with too few employees to have their own EAP sometimes use EAP services attached to private health schemes. Occupational health, counselling and advice can all be provided in this way. This solution is often the choice of charitable organisations that have small groups of employees and voluntary workers in a wide range of locations.

Telephone and Internet counselling

Face-to-face counselling is not the only format. For workers who are pressed for time or who cannot commit to regular appointments within office hours, telephone or Internet counselling is often a valuable additional resource. Shift workers or those who travel widely can access services wherever they happen to be if they have a telephone or computer connection.

A client nearly always makes first contact with a helping agency by telephone. It is beneficial if she can immediately speak to a counsellor, as she then receives empathy and understanding of her concerns without delay. The counsellors who take the calls need training to enable them to handle the unpredictable workload, to deal with highly distressed clients on the telephone and to make an assessment of the situation. A telephone counsellor has to be able to decide rapidly what to do next and what help to offer. Counsellors who answer emergency calls must have their own support system and supervision, tailored to the work that they do.

Internet counselling is still at an early stage of development, but I have no doubt that it will grow. Ease and immediacy of access mean a lot to clients. Counselling via this medium cannot use the clues gained from body language, but there is a different kind of intimacy. Sometimes the anonymity of the computer enables a client to feel that she can disclose information about herself that she might be inhibited from divulging face to face. At the same time, information may be deliberately withheld or altered to give a false impression. Counsellors who work via the Internet are aware of these possibilities, and training courses are available to help them to gain experience in this new medium.

Advice service

Counsellors generally do not give advice. The counselling process is aimed at enabling clients to make their own decisions and learn from the process.

However, many counselling services and EAPs do provide factual information for clients. Leaflets containing self-help guidelines are available for a wide range of conditions. This kind of information is very useful for stress, depression, and drug- and alcohol-related problems. Information that clients can take away and use later may bridge the gap between sessions and reinforce the learning process. A client who is not quite ready to engage in counselling will receive information that enables her to make changes for herself, or that will give her time to think and decide what to do next. She may also take information away to give to other people.

EAPs may also be able to tell clients how to obtain social service benefits to which they are entitled, how to access charitable benefits and legal and financial advice, and so on. If the EAP serves a local area, information about local services for specialised or longer-term counselling should be available. The arrangements for domestic violence, sexual abuse, mediation and family services vary greatly from one place to another, so local knowledge is invaluable for these issues. Sometimes clients want information about support groups – for example, for cancer, mental health problems such as phobias, and so on. Clients who have found counselling helpful and want to find a longer-term therapist need guidance on how to find a reputable practitioner. Each EAP will have to decide what range of information it can feasibly provide, or be able to direct clients towards other services that could be of help to them.

Critical incident debriefing

Critical incident debriefing is only occasionally needed, and an EAP manager will have to decide whether or not her team can maintain the necessary skills for this. Alternatively, an external contractor could provide this service. National EAP providers can deploy specialist teams as and when they are needed.

Emergencies sometimes result in an expectation that support services must 'do something.' Emergency response teams are trained to make an assessment of priorities, even at the height of a crisis. Without this, efforts may be misdirected. The same applies to emergency counselling services. It is not always helpful to send in a debriefing team too quickly, as there is a risk of compounding the trauma of individuals by recounting the events. Victims of trauma should not feel pressurised to receive counselling. Specialist training is needed to assess which interventions are appropriate.

Many individuals who experience traumatic events at work or in other areas of their life use the normal coping strategies of peer and family support, taking breaks and recreational activities. When trauma is a regular and inevitable part of the work, for example in Accident and Emergency departments, children's services and emergency response teams, there is a risk of burnout. Managers and professional carers must be alert for this and make sure that support is available. When a whole department or group of employees experiences a traumatic event, it may be helpful to offer group support. It remains up to the individual to choose whether or not to attend such a group.

Post-traumatic stress disorder may cause recurrent and disturbing images or flashbacks of traumatic events that interfere with a person's ability to function, and often disturb sleep. It may quickly follow traumatic experiences, but often the reaction is delayed. When the memories of severely damaging experiences are pushed away and the painful emotions denied, it may be many months or even years before the trauma resurfaces. Often there is good reason for the events to be pushed away – they are too painful and distressing to face up to at the time. An individual may feel that she has dealt well enough with a traumatic incident, and could be taken by surprise when symptoms of post-traumatic stress emerge. Sometimes a new trauma, or an event that reminds the sufferer of her past trauma, may trigger overwhelming distress. Sometimes there is no obvious precipitating factor. Counsellors offer containment and a safe environment to facilitate the processing of disturbing images resulting from post-traumatic stress.

Counselling may be responsible for reawakening disturbing memories, and practitioners must be alert to this possibility. Fear of reopening the past is a legitimate anxiety for clients who are reluctant to embark on counselling. Counsellors must be able to support clients when this happens, and have recourse to their own supervision as secondary protection.

Counselling services for alcohol and drug abuse

Alcohol and drug use is so prevalent in the general population, and therefore among professional carers, that all occupational health departments and counselling services should be aware of the effect that substance abuse may have on their clients, whether or not they are part of the presenting problem. Stress, availability of drugs intended for patients, and a vulnerable personality are all risk factors for professional carers. Substance abuse in the context of health and social care was explored in 'The quest for power' in Chapter 1 (*see* page 16) and in 'Addiction' in Chapter 4 (*see* page 74).

Occupational health physicians may be involved in determining the fitness for work of professional carers who are misusing alcohol or drugs, and monitoring their recovery. Provision for addiction counselling should be made either in-house or by referral to local specialist agencies. EAP providers usually have counsellors available with training and experience in addiction.

Doctors have access to a dedicated telephone helpline and treatment service for addiction, namely the Sick Doctors Trust. This organisation was set up to provide confidential help, in recognition of the reluctance of doctors to use the normal channels of support.

Mediation

A mediation service is a great asset to staff relationships. It may be provided by a human resource department or an EAP. When disputes, bullying or discrimination occur, mediation is a resource that can be used to resolve a problem before it escalates into a full-blown complaints procedure. Both parties must be willing to engage in the mediation process, and there should be no imbalance of power between the two. The mediator is independent of either side.

A theatrical disturbance

Alice, a scrub nurse, complained to her manager that Hassim, a technician, was rude to her and would not cooperate when they were preparing patients for operations. She felt that he did not respect her professional experience. When this was put to Hassim by his manager, he made a counterclaim of racial discrimination. He thought Alice was picking on him and making unfair judgements because of his different background.

Before making a formal complaint, they both agreed to talk about their concerns with a mediator. Each was given an uninterrupted opportunity to say what was troubling them. They were then each invited to say what they would like to happen to improve matters. The mediator was meticulous in remaining even-handed and giving both individuals a fair hearing.

Alice was surprised to find that Hassim was under considerable stress, trying to adjust to life in a different culture. She began to understand that his abrupt manner was not due to any personal animosity towards her. Hassim feared racial prejudice, but agreed that he had been treated fairly. His claim of discrimination was an angry response to Alice's complaint. Later they commented that they got on well now that they understood each other better.

Once a formal complaint has been made or disciplinary action has been taken the procedures become officious and cumbersome, and the problem is much more difficult to resolve. Workers may be suspended while complaints procedures are followed, resulting in damage to their confidence and morale, and curtailment of services to patients and clients.

Experience shows that if both parties in a dispute can be brought together with a trained mediator it is often possible to reach a mutually acceptable solution. A mediator offers a model of fairness and willingness to negotiate. If mediation is unsuccessful, formal procedures come into play. If an EAP chooses to provide this service, mediation training is required, as the necessary skills are not the same as those required for counselling.

Faith and spiritual support

Hospital chaplains provided staff support long before anyone thought of occupational health or employee assistance programmes. The 1948 Health Act stated that hospital chaplains should provide spiritual support for patients and hospital staff. Spiritual leaders of all faiths continue to do this. In 1995, *The Patients' Charter* reiterated the importance of the chaplain's role in providing spiritual support for patients and staff. The NHS employs hospital chaplains, and religious leaders also work in hospitals as an extension of their role in the community. Volunteers may assist chaplains in their work.

Chaplains have access to most parts of the hospital, so they become familiar figures. When a chaplain is visible around the hospital, it is possible for a staff member to have an informal discussion, or to arrange for a longer meeting. A chaplain will often be aware of stress, and she may know which departments are troubled when counsellors behind the doors of the EAP have no idea what is going on. Workers may feel more comfortable speaking to someone who understands their religious beliefs. Chaplains use counselling skills of listening and empathy much of the time, and some become fully trained counsellors.

In many hospitals the chapel is an ecumenical space available for collective worship, private prayer and reflection for all patients, staff and visitors, regardless of their faith.

Supervision

Counsellors are familiar with the concept of clinical supervision. It is different from line management and case management. Supervision serves the purpose of monitoring professional practice and helping counsellors to remain objective. Person-centred and psychodynamic counselling result in close emotional involvement with clients that is a vital part of the healing process. However, a counsellor must always be aware of the subconscious interaction between herself and the client. The support of a supervisor helps a counsellor to contain the emotions of her clients during the counselling process. Supervision is definitely not an optional extra that is only needed by trainees, and expendable when time is taken up by more pressing matters. It is essential for reflection and evaluation of the counselling process, whether or not there seem to be any problems. The supervision process helps counsellors to maintain boundaries and to use the emotional dimension of transference and counter-transference in the counselling relationship.

Transference in the managerial relationship was explored earlier in this chapter (*see* page 92). It is also an important part of the therapeutic process in counselling. Transference occurs when emotion is perceived to be emanating from one person when in reality it belongs to another. An example of this process was given in the case of 'Work–life balance' in Chapter 4 (*see* pages 76–7). In this case, the occupational health physician was perceived by the young doctor as a male parent figure, offering clear boundaries and approval of family values. He was not actually the young man's parent. The physician may have been acting instinctively, knowing that this was the message that the young doctor needed to hear, or he may have been consciously aware of the message he conveyed. This part of the process is known as counter-transference. The counsellor who was seeing this client needed to explore with her supervisor the contrast between her non-directive interventions and the directive approach of the physician.

Another example is given in 'My work is my life' in Chapter 1 (*see* page 13). Kirsty perceived the counsellor as a mother figure who, unlike her own mother, gave her undivided attention. In this case the counsellor was well aware of the therapeutic value of providing a nurturing model of maternal attention, and used the counter-transference to good effect.

Another example of transference can be found in 'The mountain of work' in Chapter 3 (*see* page 81). Ruth felt that her manager and senior members of the department would not help her. Indeed they did not, but her distress was compounded by the fact that this was the same response she had previously received from her family. A person who had a supportive family might have had more expectation of help and might therefore have been more likely to get it. Supervision helped the counsellor in this case to explore the influence of the client's subconscious expectations on the dynamics of her relationship with her colleagues. She could then offer an alternative model that it was reasonable to expect help in dealing with an excessive workload.

Counsellors and social workers can easily get bound up in their clients' problems, especially when seemingly overwhelming emotions are involved.

Unmanageable emotions are sometimes projected on to others. For example, a social worker who is trying to help a client whose life is out of control may also start to feel panic. Her panic may then be subconsciously conveyed to the client, and the situation can easily escalate so that neither of them knows what to do. Denied or unwanted emotions such as anger or vulnerability may also be projected on to others. Health and social care workers and counsellors frequently deny their own needs, preferring to allow sick patients and needy clients to hold the problems. Supervision is vital in giving the counsellor or care worker an opportunity to examine her own feelings in a safe environment, enabling her to retain her objectivity and competence in dealing with clients. Hawkins and Shohet[13] have examined these aspects of supervision in the helping professions.

The relationship between a counsellor and her supervisor encompasses systemic working. The complex dynamics of reflection, parallel process, transference and projection are explored in the supervision process. The understanding gained from supervision is transferred, again by parallel process, to the counsellor–client system, and subsequently to the relationship between the employee and the employing organisation. Thus the benefit of supervision and counselling does not only rest with the client. It is not easy to quantify the intangible benefits of employee counselling and supervision to the organisation, so surrogate markers such as absenteeism and staff turnover may be used for this purpose.

Supervision has another meaning in terms of management. This is about keeping to the rules and doing what the contract says. Supervision in this context may imply lack of experience or a need for control. Often supervision is regarded as a management function, and nothing whatever to do with counselling or emotions. It is important to be clear which kind of supervision is under discussion, or misunderstandings can arise.

Part of the purpose of this book is to inform supervisors who may be working with counsellors in health and social care settings. They will then be able to gain a deeper understanding of the difficulties caused by the unspoken expectations of those working in health and social care settings, and to work more effectively with the particular issues of this sector.

Counsellors are themselves members of the helping professions. They may also be compulsive carers and, like other carers, they may subconsciously hope that in caring for the emotional needs of their clients they too will be cared for. Supervisors will be able to explore this aspect of the counselling process and help counsellors to get their own needs met more effectively.

Summary

There is clear evidence that there is significant workplace stress in health and social care settings. Employers have a duty of care to employees, but also, by recognising the needs of workers for support, they provide a model for a caring environment. Professional carers explicitly and implicitly expect to be cared for. If their needs are met they are able to continue to provide care for patients and clients. The needs of the service and the needs of the workers are systemically interwoven and interdependent.

The range of support services available reflects natural process. Individual awareness and self-care are the first line of defence for coping with stress. If this fails, managers, colleagues or family may offer support. Organisational support is provided in various ways, and professional carers often have a choice of services available to them. Choice is important because counselling is likely to be ineffective if a worker feels under pressure to attend counselling, or is uncomfortable with the setting. Sometimes the use of different resources reinforces the value of the message to the client.

Counsellors who are providing staff support work at the interface between professional carers and the employing organisations, and must always keep this in mind. Person-centred counsellors can easily be drawn into focusing only on the client's problems and demonising the organisation. In many cases, a successful outcome is achieved by a combination of personal growth for the client and changes to the working environment with the support of managers. Clients may need support in asking for these changes.

Clinical supervision, as distinct from managerial supervision, is essential to enable counsellors to manage the complex psychological processes that surround systemic issues. The value of counselling is enhanced when parallel process, transference and counter-transference are understood. When projection of unwanted emotions is acknowledged, clients and counsellors can work together to contain and process them.

The benefits to individuals feed back into the organisational system and often result in improved care for patients and clients of the organisation. I find that a worker who has been helped by counselling often acts as an ambassador for the counselling service. There is no better endorsement than that of a satisfied client.

The provision of staff support services has evolved over time. To begin with, services were provided in response to demand and crisis management, resulting in a piecemeal and inconsistent service. Now it is recognised that planned support is needed, but this augments rather than replaces the rich patchwork of support that existed previously. Evolutionary development of organisations in health and social care continues and, like personal development, it is a lifelong process. The process of change will go on, and we must embrace change and learn from it both as individuals and for the sake of the caring profession as a whole. Workplace counselling in health and social care helps us to do this.

References

1 Commission for Healthcare Audit and Inspection (2005) *NHS Staff Survey 2004.* Commission for Healthcare Audit and Inspection, London.
2 Borrill CS *et al.* (1998) *Stress Among Staff in NHS Trusts: final report.* Institute of Work Psychology, University of Sheffield, Sheffield.
3 Caplan RP (1994) Stress, anxiety and depression in hospital consultants, general practitioners and senior health service managers. *BMJ.* **309:** 1261–3.
4 Collings JA and Murray PJ (1996) Predictors of stress amongst social workers: an empirical study. *Br J Soc Work.* **26:** 375–87.
5 Huxley P *et al.* (2005) Stress and pressures in mental health social work: the worker speaks. *Br J Soc Work.* **35:** 1063–79.
6 Royal College of Nursing (2002) *Working Well Survey.* Royal College of Nursing, London.
7 NHS Executive (1998) *Working Together: securing a quality workforce for the NHS.* The Stationery Office, London.
8 NHS Executive (2000) *The Provision of Counselling Services for Staff in the NHS.* The Stationery Office, London.
9 *Walker v Northumberland County Council* [1995] IRLR 35.

10 McLeod J (2001) *Counselling in the Workplace: the facts.* British Association for Counselling and Psychotherapy, Rugby.
11 Nathan J (2002) Psychoanalytic theory. In: M Davies (ed.) *Blackwell Companion to Social Work.* Blackwell Publishers, Oxford.
12 Tonks A (2003) Treating generalised anxiety disorder. *BMJ.* **326:** 700–2.
13 Hawkins P and Shohet R (2000) *Supervision in the Helping Professions* (2e). Open University Press, Buckingham.

Endpiece: What next?

The theme that runs through this book is that professional carers experience a high level of work-related stress. Conscious and unconscious motivations of people who choose to become professional carers include a desire to achieve personal fulfilment and reparation for missed opportunities in childhood. These ambitions often seem to be frustrated by the culture of the organisations that employ them to deliver health and social care.

Excessive stress is uncomfortable, and the natural impulse is to try to avoid or deny it. Psychological devices for the avoidance of distress, such as ignoring the problem and pretending it belongs to someone else, are similar for individuals and organisations. When these strategies fail, attempts may be made to 'fix' the problem by imposing control.

Workers' stress may be manifested in their personal behaviour, as anxiety, depression, anger, ill health and decreased effectiveness at work. Organisations respond to stress by changes in policy, new working practices and financial control. These in turn result in further stress for employees by mirroring and amplifying the problems. It is clear that the stress cycle can become self-perpetuating.

The impulses that lie behind career choice are always likely to be complicated and to involve psychological reparation. This is about human nature and personal growth. Organisations that provide health and social care must continue to respond to the changing needs of society and to advances in knowledge. They need to grow and develop, too, so tension and stress are inevitable. If we accept this, we can start to understand how to live with and benefit from stress instead of allowing it to damage professional carers and the organisations for which they work. The unspoken contract between a professional carer and her employer that 'I will look after the patients and service users, and in return the organisation will look after me' has to change. Professional carers must get better at looking after their own needs. The primary role of provider organisations is to take care of patients and service users. If the culture of the organisations extends to expecting and permitting workers to care for themselves, and providing the means for them to do so, the end result will be a better service.

Self-awareness and managerial awareness of stress are the starting points for exploring the underlying systemic processes. Stressed workers frequently blame their problems on the organisation. On the other hand, a worker is often the symptom carrier for a dysfunctional department. Sometimes it is necessary to stand back and allow process to do its work. It is only by looking at the whole picture that creative solutions can be found. A quick fix or a panic reaction may only perpetuate the dysfunction. The unconscious sometimes forces workers to make time for reflection. I find that clients who are too stressed to work, and who take sick leave for stress-related illness, often use the time for lateral thinking.

Workplace counsellors hold the key to unblocking the systems. A counsellor who is employed to help employees, but who also has a direct or indirect contract with the employer, can take an overview of the dynamics of the professional carer's relationship with her work. It may seem that she is serving two masters, and some find this difficult. In a sense, the workplace counsellor has both the employee and the organisation system as her client.

A counsellor may explore the parallel processes, transference and projection, that are taking place, and use this understanding to help her client to make changes if she wants to do so. Often the understanding of psychological process is not explicitly spelt out, but the counsellor's behaviour and attitude convey an alternative model of relating. When managers realise that systemic problems need to be addressed as well as individual ones, improvement may be dramatic. Sometimes clients want help to enable them to ask for systemic changes that will reduce the likelihood of a recurrence of the problem.

The relationship between a counsellor and her supervisor is vital to the process of understanding the psychodynamics of systems, as further parallel enactment also takes place in the context of clinical supervision. Supervision is an indispensable link in the counselling process. Without it a counsellor may also become drawn into a collusion that inhibits change. Many professional carers who are not counsellors would also benefit from clinical supervision, as opposed to line-managerial supervision. Doctors, nurses, personal carers and social workers are all vulnerable to the hooks of compulsive caring and the drama triangle, and may need help to stand back and take a look at their own involvement. I find that some doctors and nurses are beginning to be more aware, and professional organisations such as the British Medical Association and the Royal College of Nursing provide helpful guidance and support. My research indicates that social workers are often poorly supported by their managers and employers, and sometimes suffer from a negative public image, despite the dedication and commitment that they bring to improving the lives of their clients. Nevertheless, there are well-informed social workers who are influential in trying to change this situation, so there is optimism for the future.

Finally, I would point out that we should also remember that the glass is half full as well as half empty. The surveys that show how much damage is caused by stress among professional carers are often designed to promote campaigns to improve resources for staff support. The statistics also show that there are many professional carers who are fulfilled and happy in their work. Most carers develop personal and mutual support systems that enable them to carry on with their important work. When they need help, staff support services are usually available. Professional carers who have already received help from counselling services are quick to recommend their peers to do the same. My hope is that by writing this book I will enable those who work in health and social care to continue to grow, and that support services will go on evolving to help them to do this.

Sources of information

Agenda for Change
Department of Health
Richmond House
Whitehall
London SW1
Website: www.dh.gov.uk

Association for Counselling at Work
British Association for Counselling and Psychotherapy
BACP House
35–37 Albert Street
Rugby CV21 2SG
Website: www.bacp.co.uk

British Association for Counselling and Psychotherapy
BACP House
35–37 Albert Street
Rugby CV21 2SG
Website: www.bacp.co.uk

British Association of Social Workers
16 Kent Street
Birmingham B5 6RD
Website: www.basw.co.uk

British Medical Association
BMA House
Tavistock Square
London W1H 9JP
Website: www.bma.org.uk

Care Standards Act 2000 (Commencement No. 10 (England) and Transitional, Savings and Amendment Provisions) Order 2001, published by The Stationery Office, London.

Charity Commission
Harmsworth House
13–15 Bouverie Street
London EC4Y 8DP
Website: www.charity-commission.gov.uk

Children Act 2004, published by The Stationery Office, London.

Department of Health (2002) *Mental Health and Employment in the NHS.* Department of Health, London.

Disability Discrimination Act 1995 (c50), published by The Stationery Office, London.

Doctors Support Network for Doctors with Mental Illness
38 Harwood Road
Fulham
London SW6 4PH
Tel: 0870 321 0642
Website: www.dsn.org.uk

Employee Assistance Professionals Association (UK)
3 Moors Close
Ducklington
Witney OX29 7TW
Website: www.eapa.org.uk

Faculty of Healthcare Counselling and Psychotherapy
British Association for Counselling and Psychotherapy
BACP House
35–37 Albert Street
Rugby CV21 2SG
Website: www.bacp.co.uk

Faculty of Occupational Medicine of the Royal College of Physicians
11 St Andrews Place
Regents Park
London NW1 4LE
Website: www.rcplondon.ac.uk

General Medical Council
Regent's Place
350 Euston Road
London NW1 3JN
Website: www.gmc-uk.org

Health Professions Council
Park House
184 Kennington Park Road
London SE11 4BU
Website: www.hpc-uk.org

Investors in People UK
7–10 Chandos Street
London W1G 9DQ
Website: www.investorsinpeople.co.uk

National Institute for Health and Clinical Excellence (NICE)
MidCity Place
71 High Holborn
London WC1V 6NA
Website: www.nice.org.uk

Office for National Statistics
Room1.015
Office for National Statistics
Cardiff Road
Newport NP10 8XG
Website: www.statistics.gov.uk

Relate
Herbert Gray College
Little Church Street
Rugby CV21 3AP
Website: www.relate.org.uk

Royal College of Psychiatrists
17 Belgrave Square
London SW1X 8PG
Website: www.rcpsych.ac.uk

Sick Doctors Trust
36 Wick Crescent
Bristol BS4 4HG
Tel: 0870 4445163
Website: www.sick-doctors-trust.co.uk

United Kingdom Council for Psychotherapy
Second Floor, Edward House
2 Wakley Street
London EC1V 7LT
Website: www.psychotherapy.org.uk

UK Register of Counsellors (BACP)
Website: www.ukrconline.org.uk

Women in Surgical Training (WIST)
Royal College of Surgeons
35–43 Lincoln's Inn Fields
London WC2A 3PE
Website: www.rcseng.ac.uk

Index